The Super-Easy Dash Diet Recipes Collection for Meat Lovers

Boost Your Health with Fast and Easy Dash Recipes Affordable for Beginners

Naomi Hudson

Table of contents

Chicken Bruschetta

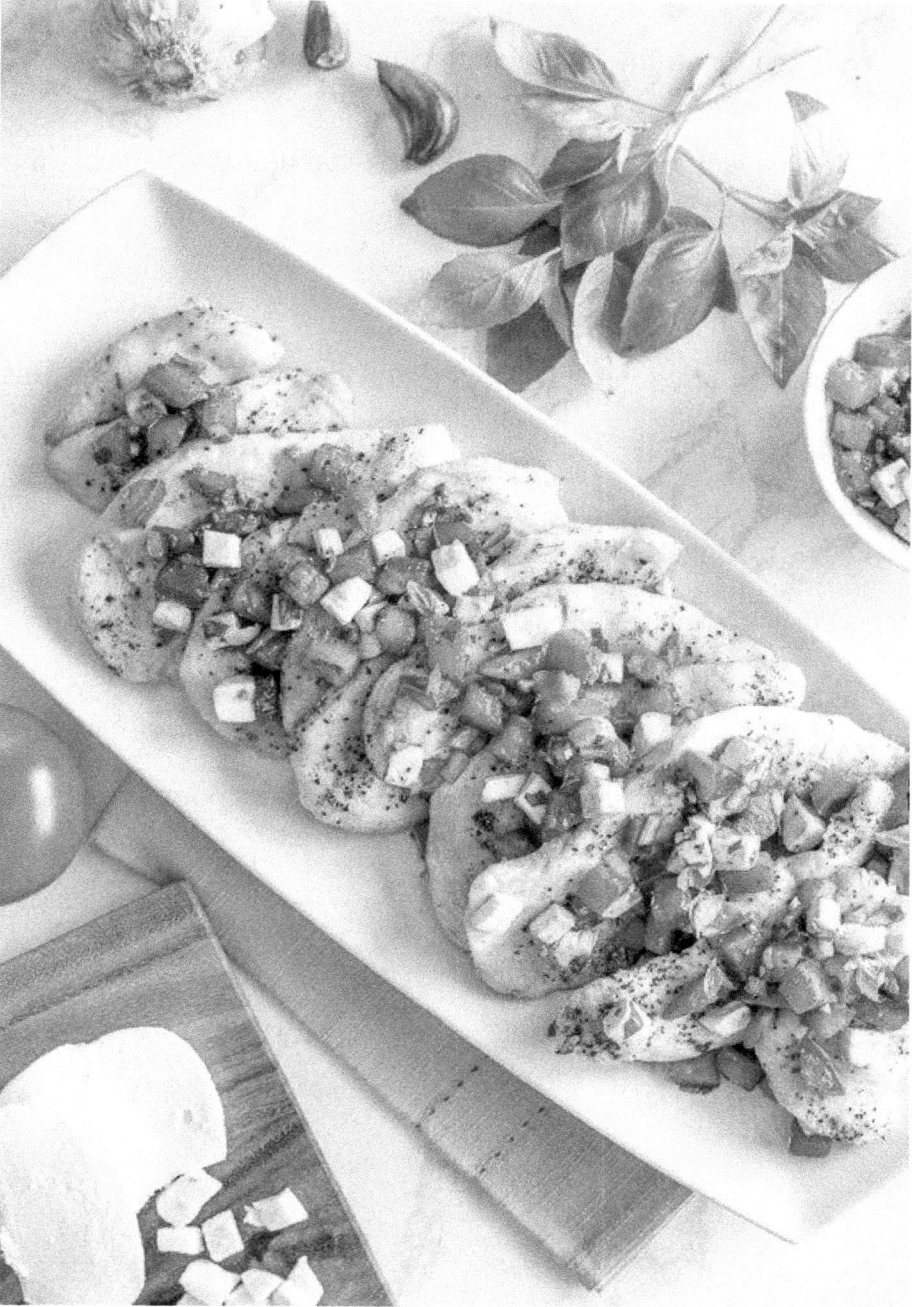

SmartPoints value: Green plan - 1SP, Blue plan - 1SP, Purple plan - 1SP

Total Time: 20 min, Prep time: 10 min, Cooking time: 10 min, Serves: 4

Nutritional value: Calories - 187, Carbs – 4.4g, Fat - 7g, Protein – 27.3g

When the weather is heating up, I mostly crave for fresh and light meals other than rich and comforting.

My most recently found new love when it comes to dessert is this deliciously prepared Italian Chicken Bruschetta. It's just so simple, simply made with

fresh tomatoes, basil, and garlic. I've tried it several times, and one sweet thing about it is the refreshing flavors. There is just something about the way the fresh and juicy tomato works together with the bright basil and bold garlic.

While preparing, I like to add some grilled chicken breast to it as a lean protein. If you've noticed, I do more of chicken breast, yes, because it is low in points, and it's a perfect way of adding protein to my meal without getting over budget with my points.

Ingredients

- Chicken breast (skinless, boneless) - 1 lb

- Large Roma tomatoes (finely diced) - 2 pieces

- Basil (finely chopped, fresh) - 1/4 cup

- Garlic (minced) - 2 cloves

- Olive oil (1 tbsp plus 1 tsp)

- Balsamic Vinegar (1/2 tsp)

- Parsley (dried) - 1 tsp

- Oregano (dried) - 1 tsp

- Pepper and Salt to taste

Instructions

1.   After cutting the chicken breasts into four equal-sized fillets, season each of the side of the chicken with the parsley, oregano and salt and pepper.
2.   Over medium-high heat, heat one teaspoon of olive oil in a medium-sized, nonstick skillet. For 4-5 minutes, cook as you turn each side until the chicken is entirely cooked and browned.

3.   Remove from heat and cover with a lid to allow it to sit for about 5 minutes.

4.   Make bruschetta by mixing tomatoes, olive oil, garlic, basil, balsamic vinegar, and pepper and salt in a bowl.

5.   Put the chicken breast on a plate and top each of them with about ¼ cup of the bruschetta. Then drizzle on some extra balsamic if you so desire.

6.   You can also make a sandwich with fresh Italian bread and little creamy goat cheese. The flavor is so bold and mouthwatering.

Lemon Chicken with Broccoli

SmartPoints value: Green plan - 3SP, Blue plan - 1SP, Purple plan - 1SP

Total Time: 30 min, Prep time: 15 min, Cooking time: 15 min, Serves: 4

Nutritional value:

Calories - 176.6, Carbs - 8.4g, Fat - 2.0g, Protein - 32.3g

The whole family will love this fantastic weeknight dinner, and it's ready in just 30 minutes. To ensure that the chicken cooks quickly and evenly, you should slice it thinly. Cover the pan when cooking the broccoli to help build up steam, bathing the florets with heat. It will allow tops that aren't in contact with the hot pan to cook properly. You will need one small to medium head of broccoli to get enough florets and one lemon to yield enough zest and juice for this entrée.

Ingredients

- All-purpose flour - 2 Tbsp

- Black pepper - ¼ tsp (freshly ground)

- Fat-free, reduced-sodium chicken broth - 1½ cup(s) (divided)

- Fresh lemon juice - 1 Tbsp

- Fresh parsley - 2 Tbsp (chopped)

- Lemon zest - 2 tsp, or more to taste*

- Minced Garlic - 2 tsp

- Olive oil - 2 tsp

- Table salt - ½ tsp (divided)

- Uncooked chicken breast(s) -12 oz, thinly sliced (boneless, skinless)

- Uncooked broccoli - 2½ cup(s), small florets Instructions

1.   On a clean plate, mix 1 1/2 Tbsp of flour, 1/4 tsp of salt, and pepper, then add chicken and turn to coat.

2.   Put a large nonstick skillet over medium-high heat and pour the oil

in for heating.

3.   Add the chicken and cook, turning as needed, until it is lightly browned and cooked through, about 5 minutes; remove to a plate.

4.   Put one cup of broth and Garlic in the same skillet, then boil over high heat, scraping up browned bits from the bottom of the pan with a wooden spoon.

5.   Add the broccoli, then cover and cook for 1 minute.

6.   Stir the remaining 1/2 cup broth, 1/2 Tbsp flour, and 1/4 tsp salt together in a small cup, then add to the skillet and bring its content to a simmer over low heat.

7.   Cover the skillet and cook until the broccoli is crisp-tender and the sauce thickens slightly.

8.   Stir in the chicken and lemon zest, then heat through.

9.   Remove the skillet from heat, and stir in the parsley and lemon juice, then toss to coat.

Chicken and Fennel in Rosemary-wine Broth

SmartPoints value: Green plan - 4SP, Blue plan - 2SP, Purple plan - 2SP

Total Time: 40 min, Prep time: 18 min, Cooking time: 22 min, Serves: 4

Nutritional value: Calories - 121.5, Carbs - 10.5g, Fat - 6.3g, Protein - 26.0g

If you are looking for a dish that will tickle your belly on a chilly night, this rustic Italian entrée is perfect, and since you will cook it in one skillet, that makes it easy to fix in your vegetable. You should first sear the chicken to produce an excellent brown exterior. You can then sauté the fennel and onion in the flavorful drippings left in the skillet. They will mix and become sweetened as they cook.

Return the chicken and any accumulated juices to the skillet to finish cooking.

Ingredients

- All-purpose flour - 5 tsp (divided)

- Black pepper - ⅛ tsp, or to taste (freshly ground)

- Canned chicken broth - 14½ oz

- Minced Garlic - 2 tsp

- Olive oil - 1 Tbsp, extra-virgin (divided)

- Red/white wine - 1/4 cup

- Rosemary - 1¼ tsp, fresh (chopped)

- Table salt - ½ tsp, or to taste

- Uncooked chicken breast(s) - 1 pound(s), cut into bite-size chunks (boneless, skinless)

- Uncooked fennel bulb(s) - 1 pound(s)

- Uncooked red onion(s) - 1 small (chopped)

Instructions

1.   Trim the stalk from fennel to quarter bulb(s) lengthwise and then slice in a cross-like manner into small pieces. Reserve the fronds for garnish (about 3 cups fennel will be available).

2.   Put the chicken on a plate and sprinkle it with rosemary, then sprinkle it with 4 tsp flour and toss to coat.

3.   Add 1 tsp of oil to a large nonstick skillet and heat over medium-high heat.

4.   Add the chicken and cook, occasionally turning with tongs, until it is lightly brown.

5.   Transfer the chicken to a clean plate (cooking is partial at this point).

6.   Heat the remaining 2 tsp oil in the same skillet over medium-high heat and add fennel and onion; sauté until it becomes lightly brown and almost tender.

7.   Add wine and Garlic, then reduce the heat to low and simmer, stirring the bottom of the pan to scrape up browned bits, until most of the wine has evaporated.

8.   Stir the broth together with the remaining 1 tsp flour in a small bowl and then stir into skillet.

9.   Add salt and pepper, then increase the heat to high and bring it to a

boil. Reduce the heat to medium-low and simmer for another 1 minute.

10.   Add the chicken and cook, often tossing until the chicken cooks through. Garnish with reserved chopped fennel fronds and serve.

You can serve it with crusty whole-grain bread, or over rice, to mop up all of the broth.

If you prefer not to use wine in this recipe, you can substitute with one tablespoon of red or white wine vinegar and three tablespoons of water.

Chicken Cordon Bleu

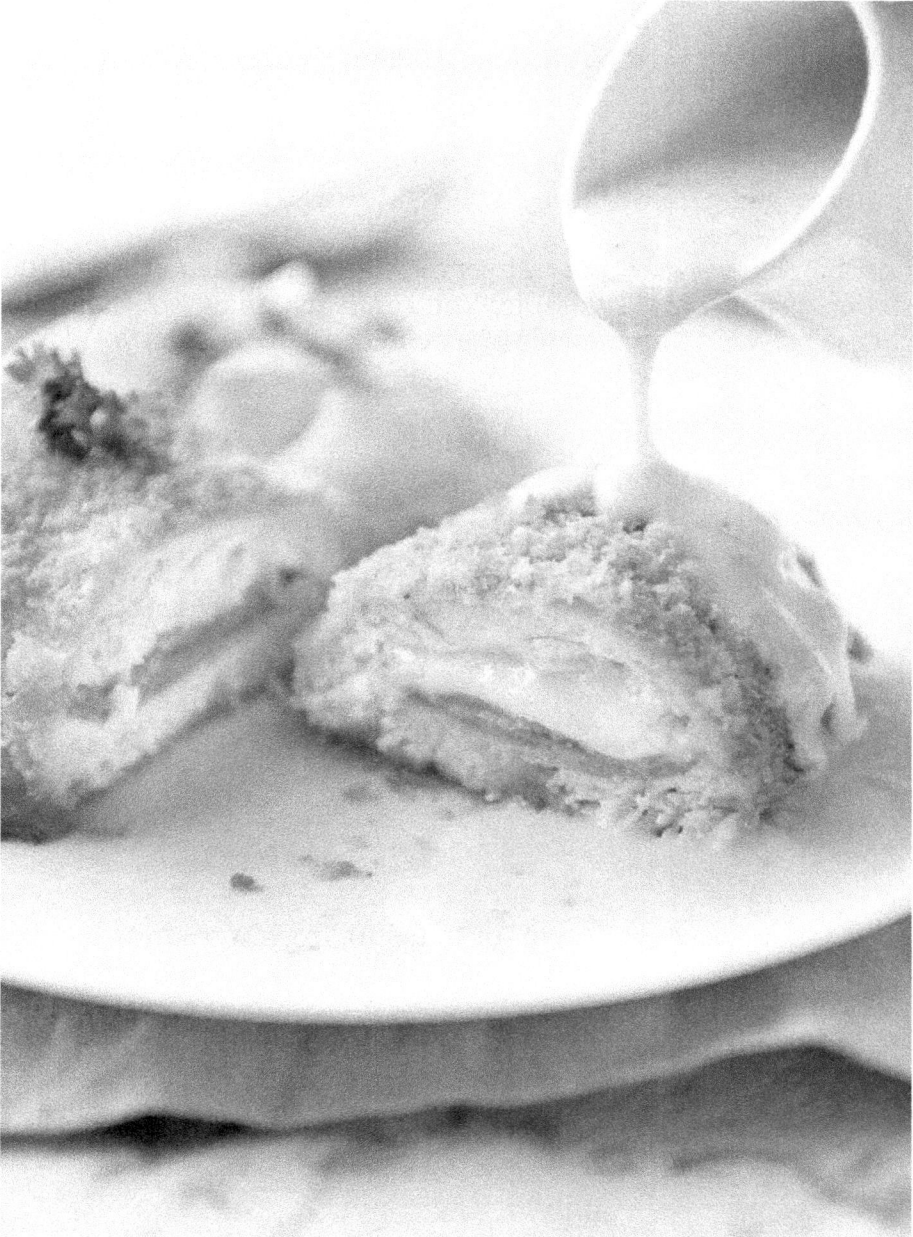

SmartPoints value: Green plan - 6SP, Blue plan - 4SP, Purple plan - 4SP

Total Time: 46 min, Prep time: 11 min, Cooking time: 35 min, Serves: 4

Nutritional value: Calories - 357.9, Carbs - 12.7g, Fat - 16.9g, Protein - 36.7g

Cordon bleu was a commonly served dish at dinner-parties in the sixties. Preparing it is simple: You sandwich a layer of ham and cheese between thin medallions of chicken or veal, then you sauté it.

Here, I have created a light version of the recipe to use a single layer of chicken rolled around the filling to make an elegant presentation.

Prepare this dish the next time you have guests and add some greens to the plate: either roasted broccolini, asparagus, or haricot vert (thin French green beans) will do just fine.

Ingredients

- All-purpose flour - 4 Tbsp

- Black pepper - ⅛ tsp (or to taste), freshly ground

- Cornflake crumbs - ½ cup(s)

- Lean ham (cooked) - 4 slice(s), (about 2 oz. total)

- Egg(s) - 1 large, lightly beaten

- Ground nutmeg - ⅛ tsp

- Parmesan cheese - 2 Tbsp, freshly grated

- Reduced-sodium chicken broth - ½ cup(s)

- Swiss cheese - 2 oz (4 thin slices), low-fat

- Table salt - ½ tsp

- Table wine - 1 Tbsp, Madeira

- Uncooked chicken breast(s) -1 pound(s), (4 breasts, 1/4 pound each), pounded to ¼-inch thickness (boneless, skinless)

- 2% reduced-fat milk - ½ cup(s)

Instructions

1.   Spray a baking sheet with nonstick spray while you preheat the oven to 400°F.

2.   Place one half of a chicken breast on a work surface and top it with one slice of the ham, then one slice of the Swiss cheese.

3.   Roll it up in a jelly-roll style, and secure with a toothpick. Repeat the process with the remaining chicken, ham, and cheese.

4.   Make a mixture of two tablespoons of flour, one-quarter teaspoon of salt, and ground pepper on a sheet of wax paper.

5.   Place the egg and the cornflake crumbs in separate shallow bowls.

6.   Taking it one at a time, coat the chicken rolls lightly, first with the flour mixture, and then dip it into the egg for a single layer coat.

7.   Coat the rolls with the cornflake crumbs, and place them on the baking sheet (discard any leftover flour mixture, egg, and cornflake bits).

8.   Spray the chicken rolls lightly with nonstick spray. Bake until the temperature of the rolls reaches 160°F, 30–35 minutes.

9.   To prepare the sauce, mix the milk, the broth, the Madeira, nutmeg, the remaining two tablespoons of flour, the remaining 1/4 teaspoon of salt, and another grinding of the pepper in a medium-sized saucepan.

10.   Whisk until it is smooth and cook over medium heat, continually whisking until it becomes thick in about 6 minutes.

11.   Remove the sauce from the heat and stir in the Parmesan cheese, then cover to keep it warm.

12.   When the chicken rolls are ready, drizzle them with the sauce and serve them immediately.

Southern-Style Oven-Fried Chicken

SmartPoints value: Green plan - 4SP, Blue Plan - 3SP, Purple plan - 3SP

Total Time: 45 min, Prep time: 15 min, Cooking time: 30 min, Serves: 4

Nutritional value: Calories - 256.9, Carbs - 31.3g, Fat - 1.6g, Protein - 27.5g

Switch to oven frying and lighten up this favorite hearty dish. I decided to improve the flavor by adding buttermilk and a pinch of cayenne pepper.

Ingredients

- All-purpose flour - ⅓ cup(s)

- Buttermilk (low-fat) - 3 oz

- Cayenne pepper - ¼ tsp (or to taste), divided

- Cooking spray - 3 spray(s)

- Cornflake crumbs - ½ cup(s)

- Table salt - ½ tsp (or to taste), divided

- Uncooked chicken breast(s) - 1 pound(s), four 4-oz pieces (boneless, skinless)

Instructions

1.   Heat the oven to 375°F before starting. Coat a 13- X 8- X 2-inch baking dish lightly with cooking spray and set it aside.

2.   Add salt and cayenne pepper to chicken for a tasty seasoning and set it aside also.

3.   Put a mixture of flour, 1/4 teaspoon salt, and 1/8 teaspoon cayenne pepper in a bowl of medium size.

4.   Put the buttermilk and cornflakes crumbs in 2 separate shallow bowls.

5.   Dip the chicken in the flour mixture and evenly coat both sides.

6.   Next, dip the flour-coated chicken into buttermilk and turn it to coat both sides.

7.   Finally, dip the coated chicken in cornflake crumbs and turn to coat both sides.

8.   Place coated chicken breasts in the baking dish that you prepared.

9.   Bake the chicken until it is tender and no longer pink in the center (you don't need to flip the chicken while baking). The baking should take about 25 to 30 minutes.

Italian Chicken Soup with Vegetables

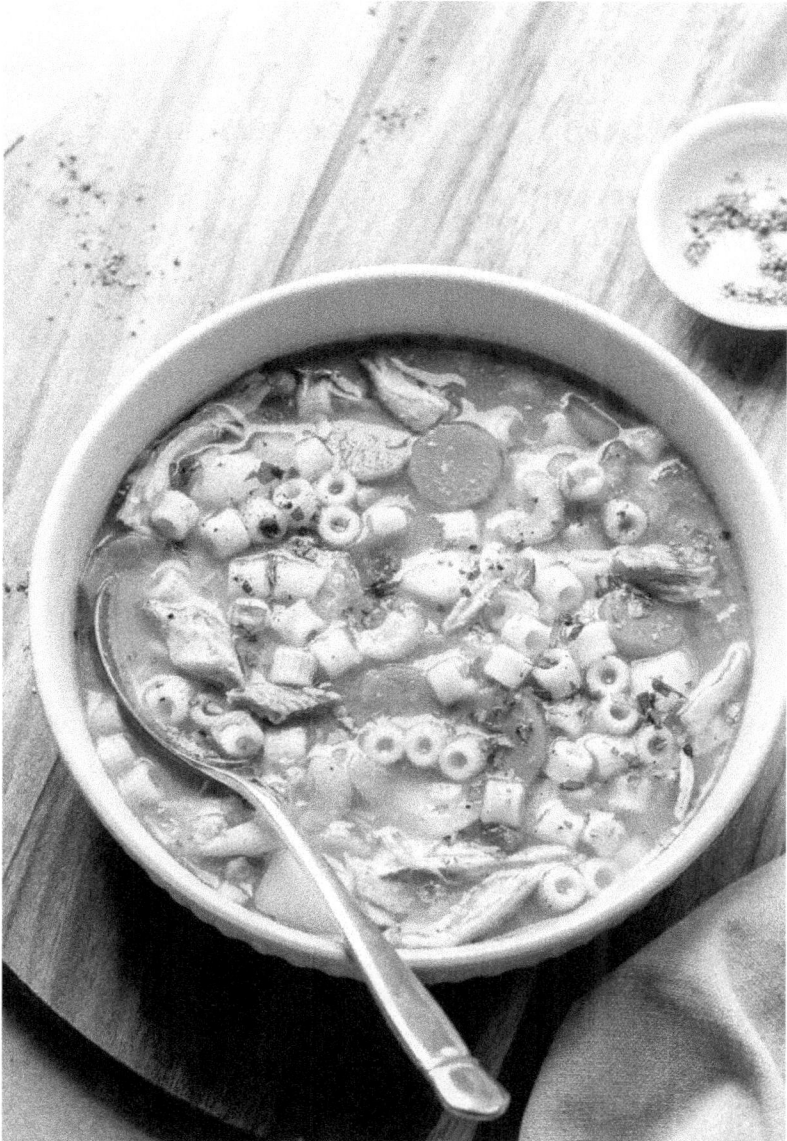

SmartPoints value: Green plan - 4SP, Blue plan - 1SP, Purple plan - 1SP

Total Time: 27 min, Prep time: 15 min, Cooking time: 12 min, Serves: 1

Nutritional value:

Calories - 136.7, Carbs - 22.3g, Fat - 1.0g, Protein - 9.6g

This chicken soup is ideal for a leisurely lunch or a quick dinner, as it is brothy and filled with vegetables. To make it bulky, you can add in any cooked grain you have on hand, like rice, barley, or quinoa, which will also add some nice texture and make it more chewable. You can use any leftover chicken you have. The drizzle of extra virgin olive oil at the end not only makes the soup look a little fancier, but it can also add a rich flavor that takes a simple soup like this one to the next level.

Ingredients

- Chicken broth - 1 cup(s), canned

- Chicken breast(s) - 1 cup(s), diced (skinless, boneless)

- Extra virgin olive oil - 1 tsp, divided

- Fresh thyme - 1¼ tsp (leaves)

- Fresh mushroom(s) - 1 cup(s), sliced

- Garlic clove(s) - 1 medium-sized, minced

- Green beans - 1 small bowl, cooked

- Lemon(s) - 1 slice(s)

- Plum tomato(es) - 1 medium-sized, diced

- Uncooked cauliflower - 1 cup(s), small florets

Instructions

1.   Heat 1/2 tsp of olive oil in a small skillet over medium heat.

2.   Add the mushrooms and garlic, then cook, continuously stirring until mushrooms begin to soften and the mixture is fragrant; about 2 minutes.

3.   Add the broth in the chicken and bring it to a boil over medium-high heat.

4.   Add cauliflower and (or) green beans, then reduce the heat to medium-low and simmer until it is almost tender; about 4 minutes.
5.   Add the chicken, thyme, and tomatoes, then simmer until the vegetables are tender; about 2 minutes.

6.   Drizzle it with the remaining 1/2 tsp of oil and fresh lemon juice, then grind the pepper over the top, if you desire.

Note: You can also garnish your dish with shredded Parmesan cheese (this could add SmartPoints values).

Roasted Chicken Breast with Spiced Cauliflower

SmartPoints value: Green plan - 4SP, Blue plan - 2SP, Purple plan - 2SP

Total Time: 50 min, Prep time: 20 min, Cooking time: 30 min, Serves: 4

Nutritional value: Calories - 470.9, Carbs - 3.5g, Fat - 11.3g, Protein - 84.2g

In this tasty recipe, you will brush chicken breasts with olive oil, turmeric, ground coriander, and cumin, with a touch of cayenne pepper before roasting, and surround it by a bed of cauliflower florets.

After cooking the chicken thoroughly, toss the cauliflower in all the delicious juices in the skillet, and let it continue to roast until it's sweet and tender. You can't have anything more convenient than a single-sheet pan dinner on a busy weeknight.

Drizzle fresh lime juice and sprinkle fresh cilantro into this Indian-influenced

meal to add incredible flavor. In case you don't like cilantro, parsley or oregano works well too.

Ingredients

- Black pepper (divided) - ½ tsp

- Cayenne pepper - ⅛ tsp

- Cooking spray - 2 spray(s)

- Cilantro (finely chopped) - 1 Tbsp
- Olive oil - 2 Tbsp

- Coriander (ground) - 1 tsp

- Turmeric (ground) - 1 tsp

- Durkee Cumin (ground) - ½ tsp

- Kosher salt (divided) - ¾ tsp

- Uncooked chicken breast - 1 pound(s), two 8 oz pieces (boneless, skinless)

- Uncooked cauliflower - 1 pound(s), cut into bite-size pieces

- Fresh lime(s) - ½ medium, with wedges for serving

Instructions

1.   Before you start, heat the oven to 450°F. Get a large baking sheet and line it with parchment paper.

2.   Combine and mix oil, turmeric, coriander, cumin, 1/2 tsp of salt, 1/4 tsp of pepper, and cayenne in a large bowl.

3.   Place the chicken in the center of the prepared baking sheet and brush each piece with 1/2 tsp of oil mixture.

4.   Add cauliflower to the bowl and toss it to coat. Place the cauliflower around the chicken and lightly coat both chicken and cauliflower with cooking spray.

5.   Sprinkle the chicken with the remaining 1/4 tsp of each salt and pepper.

6.   Roast the coated chicken until it cooks through; 15-20 minutes and

let it rest.

7.   Toss the cauliflower and chicken juices in the pan, then continue roasting until browned and tender; about 10 minutes more.

8.   Add the cilantro and toss again.

9.   Thickly slice the chicken across the grain and fan over serving plates.

10.   Serve the cauliflower and chicken in each plate and squeeze 1/2 lime over the top, then serve with additional lime wedges.

Vietnamese Chicken and Veggie Bowl with Rice Noodles

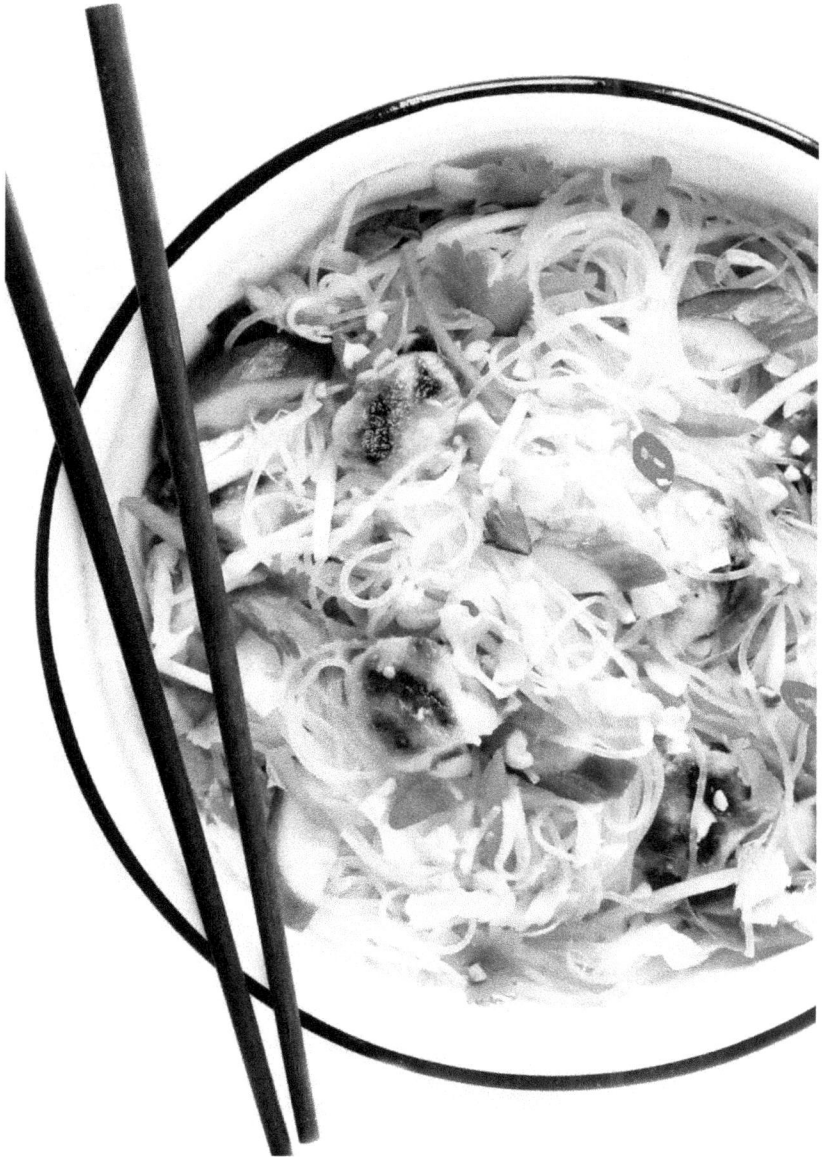

SmartPoints value: Green plan - 6SP, Blue plan - 4SP, Purple plan - 4SP

Total Time: 26 min, Prep time: 20 min, Cooking time: 6 min, Serves: 1

Nutritional value: Calories - 280.4, Carbs - 42.3g, Fat - 10.0g, Protein - 9.1g

This dish is a delicious and stunning entrée that comes together in just 25 minutes. It is a perfect recipe for one. You can even use leftover cooked chicken breast and grilled vegetables.

I would prefer you to use chicken cutlets with broccoli and red peppers, but feel free to experiment with chicken thighs, spinach, mushrooms, onions, or whatever you have on hand.

The soy and fish sauces add that ultimate umami bomb, while sriracha helps keep it balanced out by providing a touch of heat.

You can quickly scale up this recipe if you need to serve it to a crowd. Ingredients

- Cilantro (chopped, fresh leaves) - 2 Tbsp

- Cooked rice noodles - ½ cup(s)

- Asian fish sauce - ½ tsp

- Cooking spray - 4 spray(s)

- Uncooked chicken breast - 5 oz, thin cutlet (boneless, skinless)

- Uncooked broccoli - 1 cup(s), small florets or baby stalks

- Red pepper(s) (sweet) - ½ medium, cut in 2 even pieces

- Soy sauce (low sodium) - 2 Tbsp, divided (or to taste)

- Sriracha sauce - 1 tsp (or to taste)

- Sugar - ¼ tsp

- Roasted peanuts (unsalted dry) - 2 tsp, chopped

Instructions

1.   Coat a grill or grill pan with cooking spray and preheat on medium-high heat.

2.   Place the chicken, broccoli, and red pepper in a shallow bowl and drizzle with one tablespoon of soy sauce, then toss to coat.

3.   Coat the chicken with cooking spray and grill, turning the chicken once and the vegetables a few times, until chicken cooks through and veggies are tender-crisp; about 6 minutes.

4.   Slice the chicken and pepper them into strips, then place all in a bowl over noodles.

5.   Stir together the remaining one tablespoon of soy sauce, fish sauce, and sugar. Drizzle the mixture over your cooked chicken.

6.   Sprinkle a mixture of cilantro, peanuts, and sriracha on the chicken, then serve.

Chicken Tortilla Soup

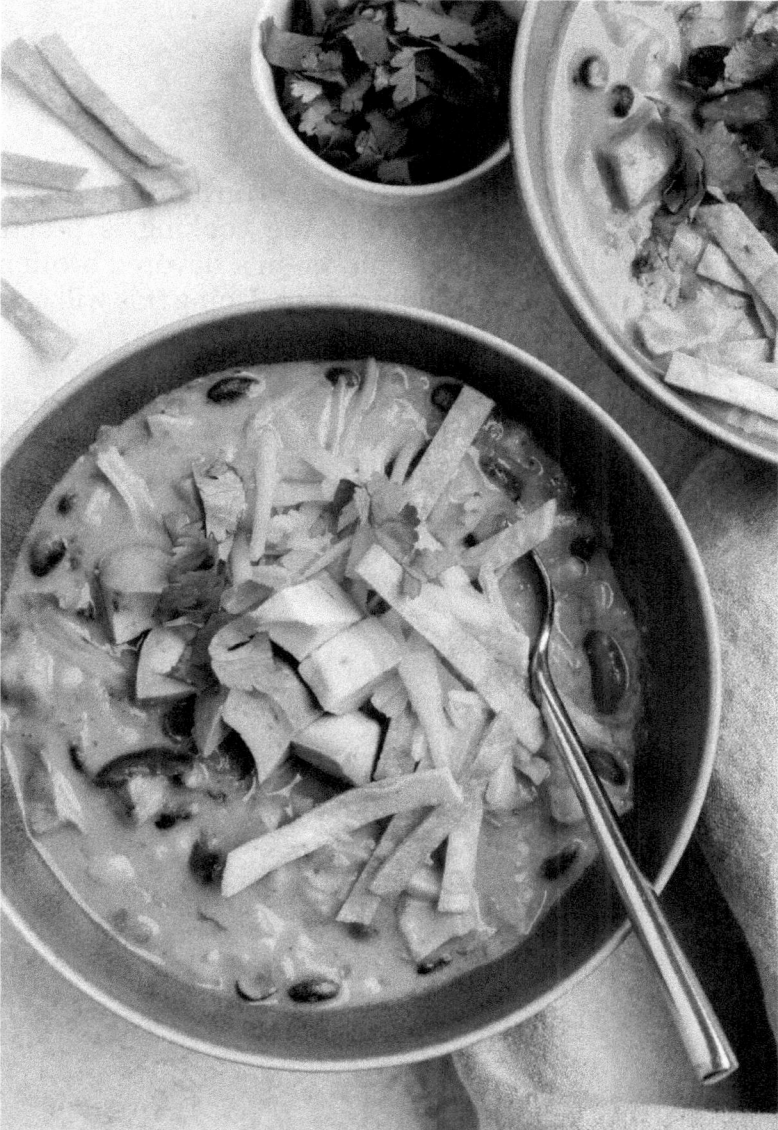

SmartPoints value: Green plan - 4SP, Blue plan - 2SP, Purple plan - 2SP

Total Time: 45 min, Prep time: 15 min, Cooking time: 30 min, Serves: 6

Nutritional value:

Calories - 200, Carbs - 24g, Fat - 9g, Protein - 7g

Preparing this soup is very easy. Once you have chopped and sautéed the vegetables, the rest of the cooking is practically hands-off. You will simmer the chicken in a flavored broth made with fire-roasted tomatoes and lime juice. Doing this will give you some extra minutes to put together a quick

salad or other simple side dishes. Chicken breasts (boneless, skinless) work well in this soup, but you can use chicken thighs as well. If you'd like to make things more interesting, don't de-seed the jalapeño completely.

Ingredients

- Cilantro (chopped) - 1 cup(s)

- Chili powder - 1 tsp

- Chicken broth (reduced-sodium) - 6 cup(s)

- Olive oil - 1 tsp

- Uncooked onion(s) (chopped) - 1½ cup(s)

- Kosher salt -1½ tsp

- Minced Garlic - 4 tsp

- Jalapeño pepper(s) - 1 medium (seeded and minced)

- Tomatoes (canned, diced)- 15 oz, fire roasted-variety, drained

- Uncooked chicken breast - 20 oz (boneless, skinless)

- Lime juice (fresh) - ⅓ cup(s)

- Mexican-style cheese (Shredded reduced) - 6 Tbsp

- Tortilla chips (crushed) - 12 chip(s)

Instructions

1.   Set a soup pot over medium heat and preheat.

2.   Toss in the chopped onion and salt, then cook, often stirring, until the onion gets soft; 5-10 minutes.

3.   Add garlic, chili powder, and jalapeno, then cook for one minute.

4.   Put in your broth, tomatoes, lime juice, and chicken, then stir to combine.

5.   Simmer and cook until the chicken breasts cook through; about 20 minutes.

6.   Remove the chicken breasts from the soup and shred them with two forks, then return the shredded chicken to the pot with cilantro.

7.   Serve your soup garnished with tortilla chips and cheese.

Chicken Piccata Stir-Fry

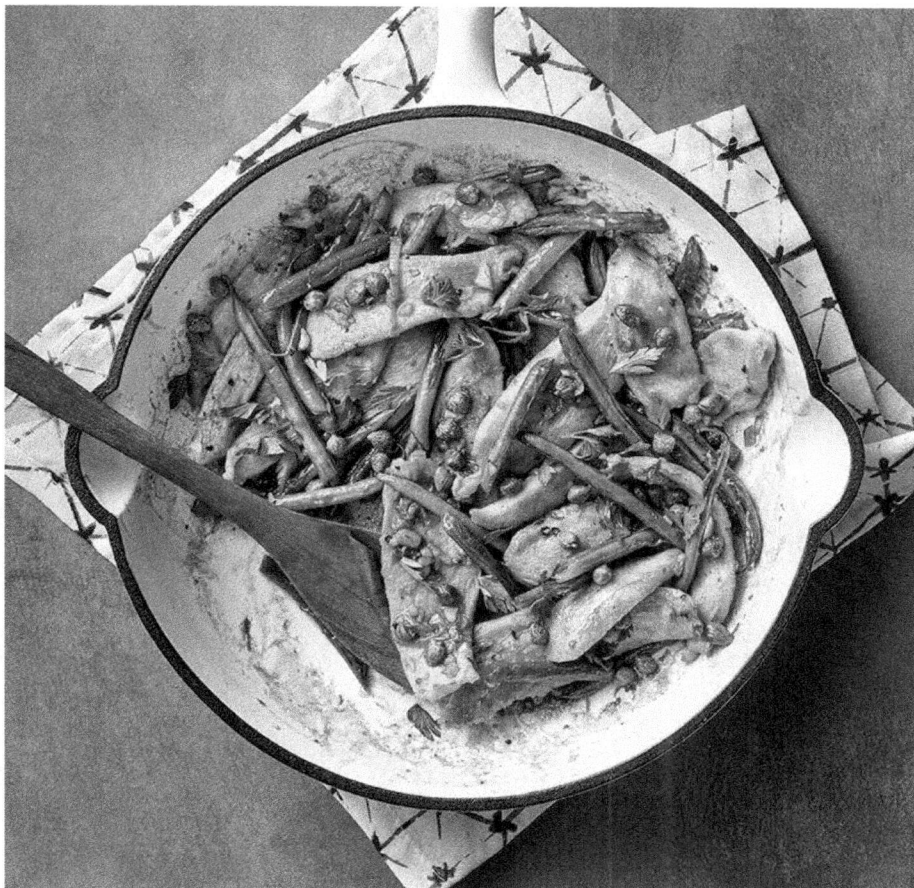

SmartPoints value: Green plan - 4SP, Blue plan - 2SP, Purple plan - 2SP

Total Time: 25 min, Prep time: 20 min, Cooking time: 5 min, Serves: 4

Nutritional value: Cal - 190.5, Carbs - 5.6g, Fat - 9.4g, Protein - 18.6g

This dish is a combination of the classic Italian chicken piccata and Asian stir-fry.

Ingredients

- Black pepper (freshly ground) - ¼ tsp

- Capers (rinsed)- 1 Tbsp

- Chicken broth (fat-free) - ½ cup(s)

- Cornstarch (divided) - 2 tsp

- Dry sherry (divided)- 3 Tbsp

- Table salt (divided) - ¾ tsp

- Soy sauce (low sodium) - 1 Tbsp

- Peanut oil (divided) - 4 tsp, or vegetable oil

- Uncooked chicken breast (boneless, skinless) - 1 pound(s), cut into quarter-inch-thick slices

- Uncooked shallot(s) - 1 medium, thinly sliced Minced Garlic - 1 Tbsp

- String beans (uncooked) - 2 cup(s), cut into two-inch lengths Parsley (fresh, chopped) - 2 Tbsp

- Lemon(s) - ½ medium, cut into four Instructions

1.   Prepare a clean medium-sized bowl and mix chicken, 1 tsp of cornstarch,1 Tbsp of dry sherry,1/2 tsp salt, and pepper in it.

2.   Next, get a small bowl and combine broth, soy sauce, remaining 2 Tbsp of dry sherry, and 1 tsp of cornstarch.

3.   Preheat a fourteen-inch flat-bottomed wok or twelve-inch skillet

over high heat to the point where a drop of water will evaporate within 1 to 2 seconds of contact, then swirl in one Tbsp oil.

4.   Add shallots and garlic, then stir-fry for 10 seconds. Push the shallot mixture to the sides of the wok and add the chicken, then spread in one layer in the wok.

5.   Cook the chicken undisturbed for 60 seconds, allowing the chicken to begin searing, then stir-fry another 60 seconds until chicken is no longer pink but not yet thoroughly cooked.

6.   Swirl the chicken in the remaining 1 tsp oil and toss in green beans and capers. Sprinkle on the remaining 1/4 tsp of salt and stir-fry for 30 seconds or until just combined.

7.   Swirl the chicken in the broth mixture and stir-fry for 1-2 minutes or until the chicken is cooked through, with the sauce slightly thickened.

8.   Sprinkle the parsley on it and serve with lemon wedges.

Ranch Meatballs

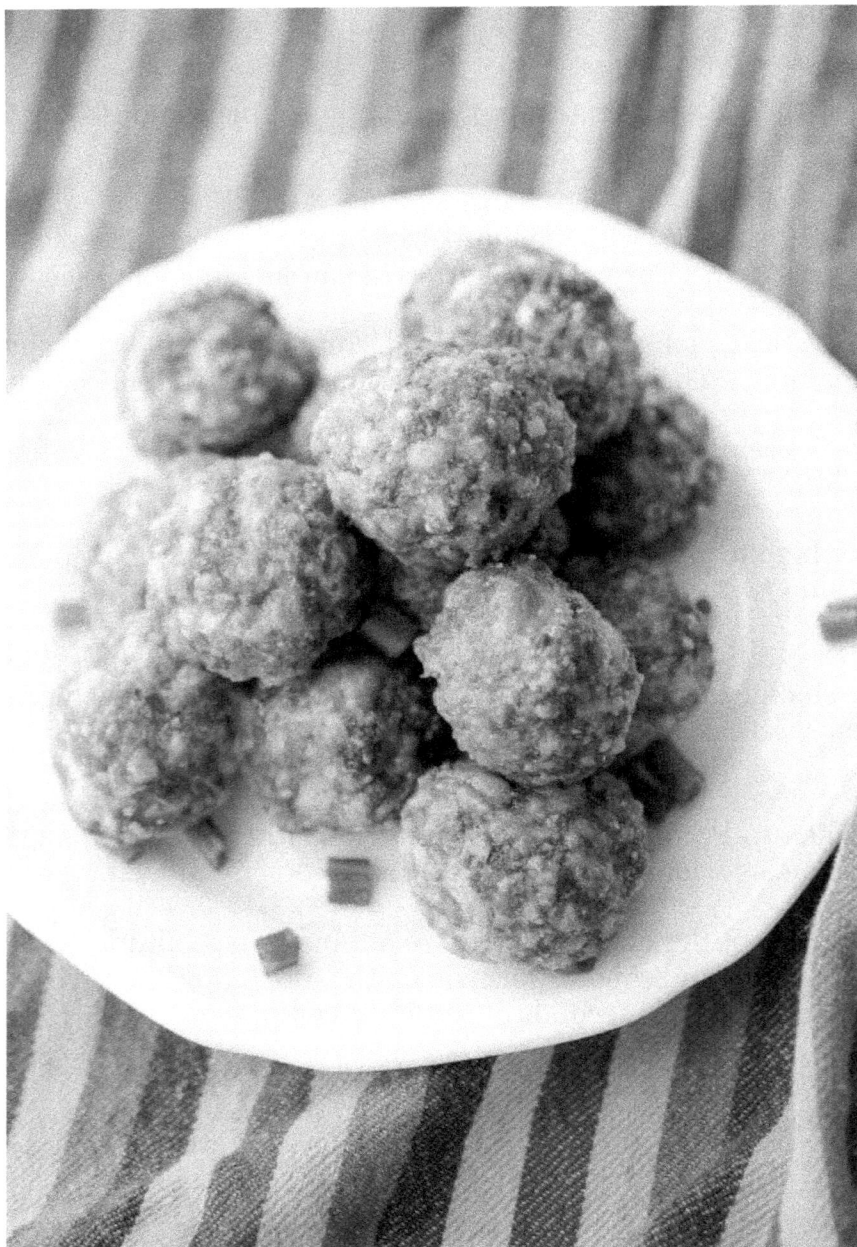

SmartPoints value: Green plan - 4SP, Blue plan - 4SP, Purple plan – 5SP

Total Time: 20mins, Prep time: 10 mins, Cooking time: 30mins, Serves: 4

Nutritional value: Calories - 195, Carbs - 6g, Fat - 6g, Protein - 26g

Meatball recipes are delicious protein recipes that are so satisfying and tasty. They can be a fun and easy meal. It becomes easier to prepare the perfect sized meatballs using a meatball shaper.

Ingredients

- Ground beef (96/4) (extra lean) - 1 lb

- Panko breadcrumbs - 1/3 cup(s)

- Egg substitute (Liquid, like egg beaters) - 1/4 cup

- Olive oil - 1 tsp

- Onion powder - 1 tbsp

- Garlic powder - 1 tbsp

- Dill (dried) - 2 tsp

- Parsley (dried) - 2 tsp

- Basil (dried) - 2 tsp

- Salt and pepper - Add to taste

Instructions

1.   Combine all the ingredients by hand in a large bowl and shape it into about 24 meatballs.

2.   Apply heat to the oil in a large non-stick skillet over medium-high heat.
3.   Place meatballs in the pan and cook for about 1-2 minutes on each side, until all sides get lightly browned.
4.   Reduce the heat to medium-low and pour in half a cup of water. Cover it and cook, occasionally stirring, until meatballs cook thoroughly; about 10-12 minutes.

Note: Meatballs are a perfect simple Weight Watchers dinner recipe for those who are watching Points but also savour the flavour

Beef Orzo with Feta

SmartPoints value: Green plan - 8SP, Blue plan - 8SP, Purple plan – 8SP

Total Time: 35mins, Prep time: 10mins, Cooking time: 25mins, Serves: 6

Nutritional value: Calories - 325, Carbs – 44g, Fat – 5.5g, Protein – 25g

Beef Orzo is one of those types of meals that you'll love to prepare now and then. The instructions for preparation are quite easy to follow, and the meal is just delicious. If you haven't tried it, you are missing out big time. You should give it a try for your next family dinner or friends gathering. This most satisfying weight-watching dinner recipe is perfect for warming you and your family up on a chilly fall evening.

Ingredients

- Ground beef (extra-lean) - 1 lb

- Whole wheat orzo - 10 oz

- Onion (finely chopped) - 1 large

- Garlic (minced) - 4 cloves

- Cinnamon (ground) - 1 tsp

- Oregano (dried) - 2 tsp

- Can tomatoes (crushed) - One 26oz

- Reduced-fat feta cheese (crumbled) - 1/3 cup

- Salt & pepper - Add to taste

Instructions

1. Prepare whole orzo wheat according to package directions. Drain it and set aside.

2. While the wheat is cooking, spray a large skillet with nonfat cooking spray, and set it over medium-high heat. Toss in some beef and cook until it mostly cooks through.

3. Put in onions, oregano, garlic, cinnamon, salt, and pepper. Sauté the dish until the onions are tender and the beef cooks all the way through.

4. Pour the crushed tomatoes into the skillet with the beef mixture, and cook on medium heat. Continue to cook, while occasionally stirring, until the mixture thickens; about 15 minutes.

5. Dish the beef sauce with orzo and place in serving bowls. Top each bowl with 1 tbsp of feta.

Light Beef Chili

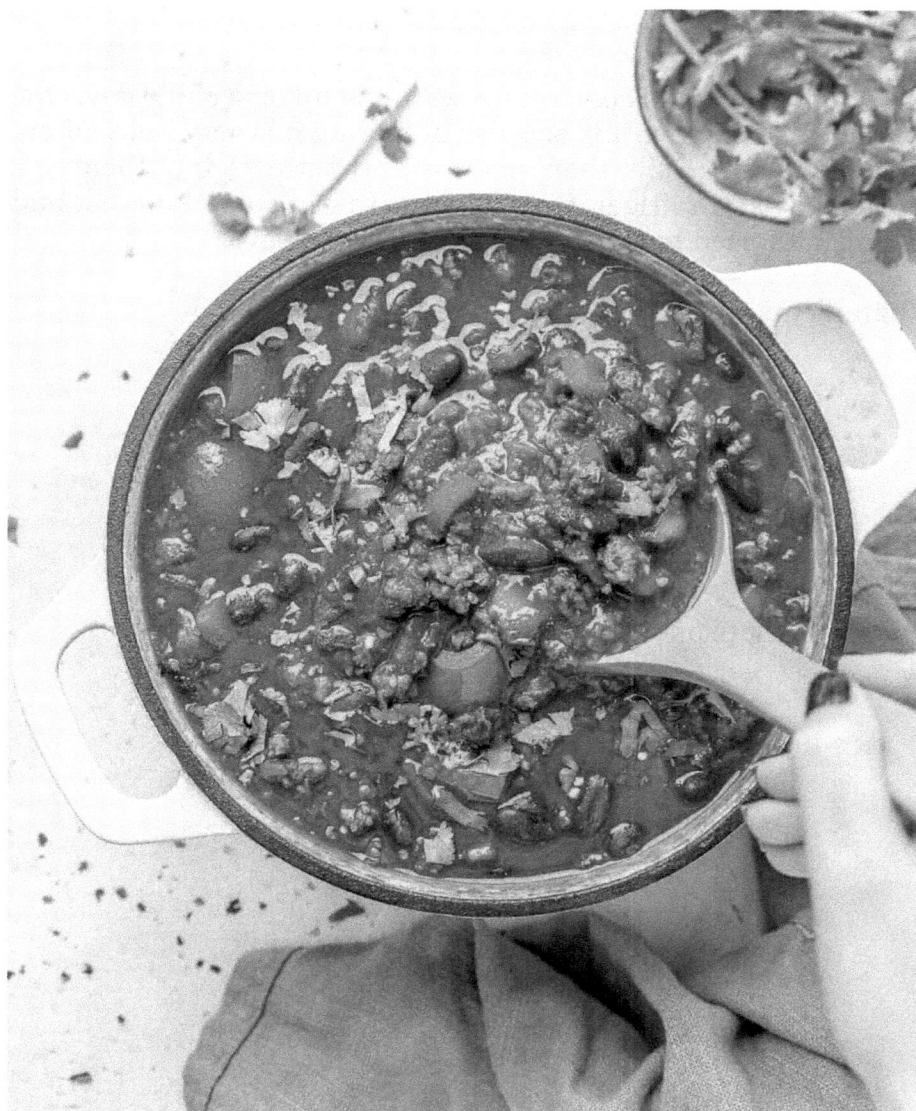

SmartPoints value: Green plan - 4SP, Blue plan - 4SP, Purple plan – 4SP

Total Time: 2hrs 30mins, Prep time: 30mins, Cooking time: 2hrs, Serves: 8

Nutritional value: Calories - 187, Carbs – 24g, Fat – 3g, Protein – 16g

This red meat dish is perfect for warming up on a chilly day. One of the reasons I love it is because preparing it is very easy. Often, I will make this chili, then measure and place each of them in a Ziploc bag and refrigerate. Whenever I need something hot and filling, all I need to do is grab one and microwave.

Ingredients

- Beef bouillon powder - 1 tbsp

- Bell pepper (red, diced) - 1 small

- Black pepper - 1/2 tsp

- Brewed coffee (strong) - 1 cup

- Chili powder - 3 tbsp

- Cocoa (unsweetened) - 1 tsp

- Cumin - 2 tbsp

- Dark beer - One 12oz can

- Garlic (minced) - 4 cloves

- Green pepper (diced) - 1 small

- Ground beef (extra lean) - 1 lb

- Kidney beans - One 15oz can

- Onion (diced) - 1 large

- Oregano - 2 tsp

- Paprika - 1 tsp

- Salt - 1 tsp

- Sugar - 1 tbsp

- Tomatoes (diced) - One 28oz can

- Tomato sauce - One 8oz can

Instructions

1.   Place a large pot or Dutch oven over medium-high heat and spray it with non-fat cooking spray.

2.   Add the onions and garlic, then cook until onions start to soften; about 3 minutes.

3.   Toss in the ground beef and cook until the meat turns brown.

4.   Add the diced bell peppers to the beef and cook for another 5 minutes.

5.   Put in all the remaining ingredients asides the kidney beans and stir.

6.   Bring the content of the pot to a simmer, then stir in the kidney beans.

7.   Reduce the heat to medium-low, cover the pot, and let it cook for about 2 hours.

This perfect hearty beef chili made with extra lean ground beef simmers in fantastic spices and flavors to give you a desirable taste.

Crudities

Nutrition

Calories: 22 kcal | Gross carbohydrates: 5 g | Protein: 1 g | Fats: 0.2 g | Fiber:

2 g | Net carbohydrates: 3 g | Macro fat: 5 % | Macro proteins: 24 % | Macro

carbohydrates: 71 %

Total time: 10 minutes

Ingredients

- 1 celery stem

- 1 bush of chicory cuts lengthwise into four pieces Cut 10 cm cucumber into long, thin strips

- 2 peppers, for example, red and yellow Instructions

1.   Cut the vegetables into thin, long strips so that you can dip them. For example, you can use chicory, little gem lettuce, cucumber, colored peppers, and celery.

2.   Tasty and fast - if you don't feel like cooking.

Herring with Onions

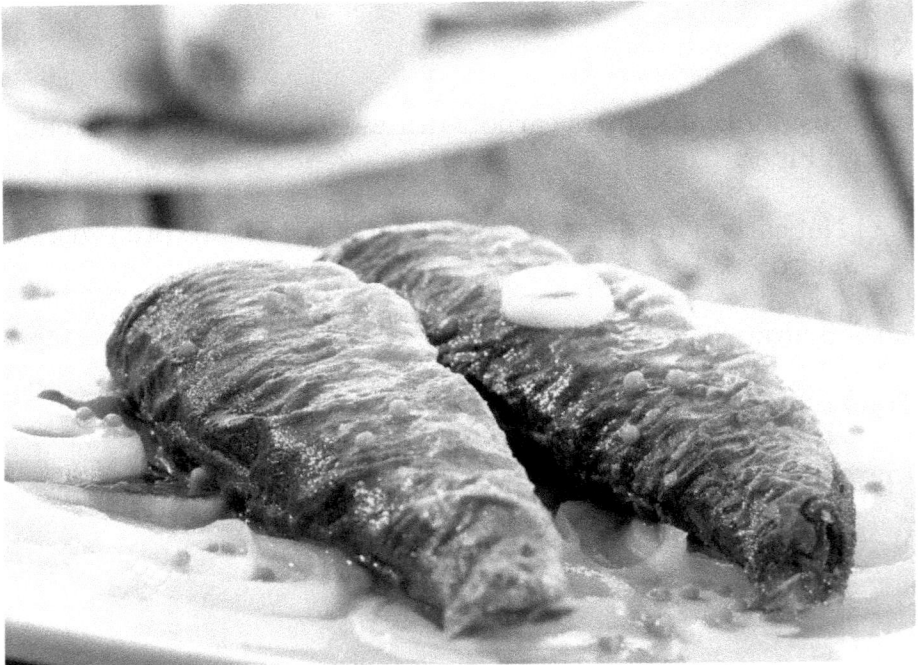

Nutrition

Calories: 111 kcal | Gross carbohydrates: 3 g | Protein: 12 g | Fats: 6 g | Fiber:

0.3 g | Net carbohydrates: 3 g | Macro fat: 29 % | Macro proteins: 58 % |

Macro carbohydrates: 13 %

Time - 15 minutes

Ingredients

- 1 haring

- 1 tablespoon onion

- Instructions

- A very quick lunch.

Notes

If you follow the keto diet, you can still get some goodies from the fish stall.

Tasty and very healthy! Herring contains many Omega 3 fatty acids.

Insalata Capricciosa

Nutrition

Calories: 551 kcal | Gross carbohydrates: 9 g | Protein: 28 g | Fats: 46 g |

Fiber: 3 g | Net carbohydrates: 6 g | Macro fats: 58 % | Macro proteins: 35 % |

Macro carbohydrates: 8 %

Time: 15 minutes

Ingredients

- 2 eggs

- 2 tomatoes around 200 grams

- 100 grams of mixed lettuce or iceberg lettuce

- 60 grams of black olives, preferably in olive oil

- 100 grams of mozzarella

- 100 grams of tuna in water or olive oil

- pepper and salt

- 50 ml extra virgin olive oil

- 15 ml of lemon juice

Instructions

1. Bring a saucepan of water to the boil. Once the water boils,

carefully lay the eggs in it. Bring the water back to the boil and boil the eggs for 8 minutes. Then place the pan under the cold tap so that the eggs cool sufficiently to allow them to peel.

2.   Wash the tomatoes, pat them dry with kitchen paper and cut into slices.
3.   Drain the tuna well and place it on top of the lettuce.
4.   Also, divide the tomato and olives slices over the lettuce and also cut the boiled eggs into slices. Put it on the lettuce too.
5.   Season the salad with salt and pepper. Make a vinaigrette by mixing the olive oil well with the lemon juice in a cup. Use a teaspoon to distribute the vinaigrette on the plates.

Oopsie sandwich (keto)

Nutrition

Calories: 84 kcal | Gross carbohydrates: 2 g | Protein: 4 g | Fats: 7 g | Fiber: 1

g | Net carbohydrates: 1 g | Macro fats: 58 % | Macro proteins: 33 % | Macro

carbohydrates: 8 %

Total time: 30 minutes

Ingredients

2 eggs

75 grams of cream cheese

1 teaspoon of psyllium

0.5 teaspoon baking powder

pinch of salt

Instructions

1.   Preheat the oven to 150° Celsius and ensure that the eggs are at room temperature. When the eggs come out of the refrigerator, place them in a bowl of lukewarm tap water for 10-15 minutes.

2.   Split the eggs. Put the egg whites in a cup for a hand blender and the egg yolks in another bowl.

3.   Mix the egg yolks with the cream cheese, the psyllium and the baking powder with a whisk or a fork. Let this batter rest for 5 minutes so that the baking powder and psyllium can work.

4.   Beat the egg whites with a pinch of salt. The proteins must be so stiff that if you hold the cup upside down, they will not move.

5.   Carefully scoop the egg whites through the egg yolk-cream cheese mixture. The mixture must become nicely airy.

6.   Put a sheet of baking paper on an oven plate and make 8 heaps of batter on the baking sheet.

7.   Bake in 25 minutes at 150° Celsius. The sandwiches must be beautifully golden brown.

Keto (gluten-free) poffertjes

Nutrition

Calories: 700 kcal | Gross carbohydrates: 8 g | Protein: 27 g | Fats: 63 g |

Fiber: 1 g | Net carbohydrates: 7 g | Macro fats: 65 % | Macro proteins: 28 % |

Macro carbohydrates: 7 %

Total time: 40 minutes

Ingredients

- Keto poffertjes

- 4 eggs

- 250 grams of ricotta

- 1 tablespoon psyllium, for example, Livinggreens psyllium fibers

- 0.5 teaspoon baking powder

- 0.25 teaspoon vanilla extract

- 2 tablespoons of mild olive oil

- Whipped cream

- 200 ml whipped cream

- 0.5 teaspoon vanilla extract

Instructions

1.	Allow the eggs to reach room temperature by removing them from the fridge 15 minutes in advance or by placing them in lukewarm tap water for 5 minutes.
2.	If you have made your own ricotta, use a hand blender or hand blender until there are no / few lumps. If you have ricotta from the store this is not necessary.

3.	Now add the ricotta, the baking powder (optional), vanilla extract and the psyllium to the beaten eggs and mix well with a fork.

4.	Let the batter stand for 5-10 minutes so that it becomes a little stronger.
5.	Heat a cast-iron poffertjes pan over high heat so that it becomes hot. Then grease the pan with a mild olive oil with a brush and lower the heat.
6.	Now place a spoonful of batter in each compartment in the pan. Make sure you have lowered the heat now!
7.	Bake the pancake for 2-4 minutes on one side (depending on how large the pancake is). When the top starts to dry, turn the poffertje with a spoon and bake the other side. Repeat until all the batter has been used up.

8.   Beat the whipped cream with the vanilla extract or use a whipped cream machine.
9.   Serve cold or hot.

Notes: Delicious with fresh raspberry or chia raspberry jam or chia blueberry jam or homemade keto-Nutella.

Frittata with Chanterelles

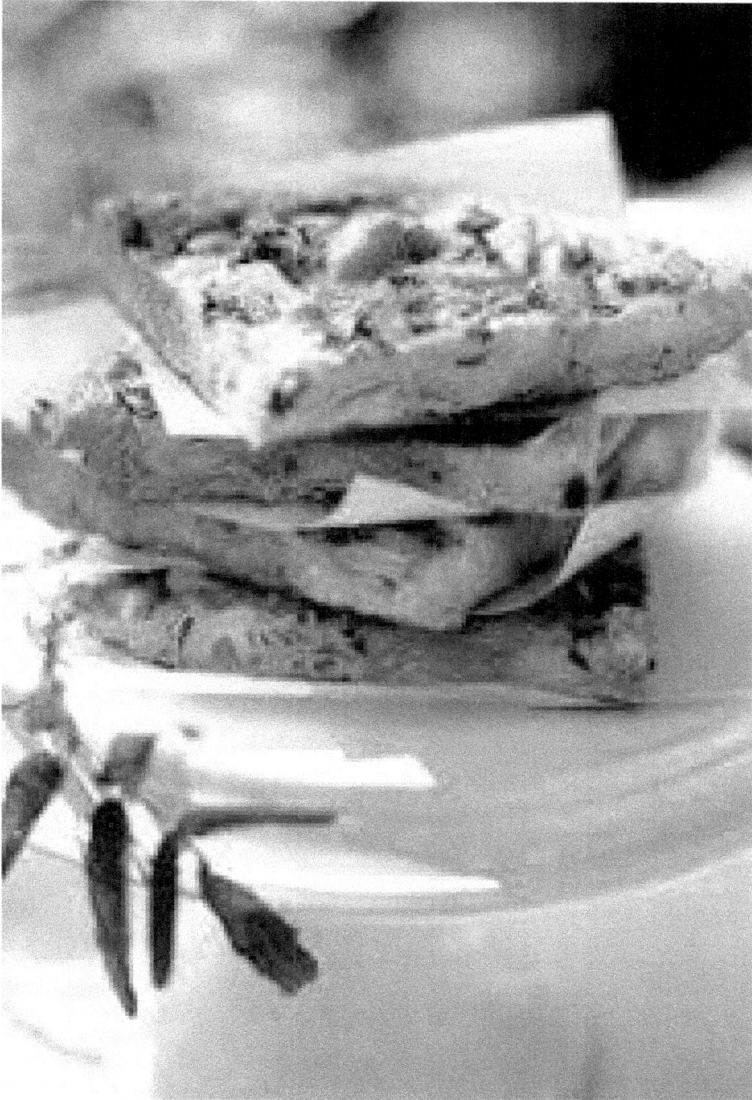

Nutrition

Calories: 1011 kcal | Gross carbohydrates: 13 g | Protein: 21 g |
Fats: 97 g |

Fiber: 4 g | Net carbohydrates: 9 g | Macro fats: 76 % | Macro proteins: 17 % |

Macro carbohydrates: 7 %

Total time: 25 minutes

Ingredients

- 6 eggs

- 250 grams of chanterelles

- 50 tablespoons butter

- 50 ml extra virgin olive oil

- 1 clove of garlic

- 1 tablespoon oregano leaves without stalk

- 1 tablespoon of young sage leaves

- 0.5 lemon

- 300 ml mascarpone

- Creme fraiche dip

- 1 forest outing

- 200 ml creme fraiche

Instructions

1.   Preheat the oven to 220° Celsius.

2.   If the eggs are not yet at room temperature, remove them from the refrigerator and place them in a bowl of warm water (not boiling!).

3.   Use a mushroom brush to gently clean the chanterelles. Leave them whole.
4.   Heat the butter with the olive oil in a frying pan. Add the chanterelles to the pan as soon as the butter has melted and bake for 3-4 minutes until medium to high heat. Turn over occasionally.

5.   Clean the garlic and chop it into small pieces.
6.   Wash the sage and oregano, pat dry and chop into small pieces.

7.   Add the garlic and spices to the skillet and turn the heat down. Cook for 4-5 minutes. Remove the pan from the heat and squeeze half a lemon over the chanterelles.
8.   Grease a baking dish and / or put a sheet of baking paper in it.

9.   Beat the eggs with the mascarpone in a bowl and add some salt and pepper.
10.   Put the chanterelles in the baking dish and pour the beaten eggs over it. Bake in the oven for 10-15 minutes, until the egg is firm.
11.   You can check whether the frittata is fully cooked by piercing it with a wooden or metal stick. If the skewer comes out clean, the frittata is ready.
12.   Clean a spring onion and cut into rings. Mix through the creme fraiche.
13.   Serve with creme fraiche.

Niçoise Salad with Tuna Steak

Nutrition

Calories: 956 kcal | Gross carbohydrates: 6 g | Protein: 37 g | Fats: 86 g |

Fiber: 2 g | Net carbohydrates: 4 g | Macro fats: 68 % | Macro proteins: 29 % |

Macro carbohydrates: 3 %

Total time: 18 minutes

Ingredients

Tuna steaks

- 375 grams of tuna steaks If you use frozen food, defrost beforehand.

- 3 tablespoons butter

- Eggs

- 3 eggs

- Vegetable

- 0.5 celeriac

- 90 grams of cherry tomatoes

- 180-gram haricot verts Drained weight - from a pot without added sugar

- 1 bunch of radishes

- 1 tablespoon capers

- 3 tablespoons olives If you buy olives in oil, make sure they are in olive oil and not in any other type of oil!

Dressing

- 300 ml mayonnaise

Instructions

1. Eggs

2. Start by boiling the eggs. Cook them in 8 minutes and then put them in a pan with cold water to cool.
3. Peel and halve the eggs.
4. Place the eggs on a large flat dish.
5. Tuna steaks
6. Melt the butter or ghee in a skillet or use a grill pan without butter.

7. Cook the tuna in 2.5 minutes per side (or until cooked, depending on the thickness of the tuna steak).
8. Place the tuna steaks on top of the haricot verts.
9. Vegetable
10. Use half a celery tuber. Cut the half tuber into 1.5

cm thick slices. Remove the skin and cut the slices into small cubes (approximately 1 cm -1.5 cm). Cook the cubes in the microwave or in a saucepan with some water. Allow to cool.

11. Drain the haricot verts and then place them in the middle of the serving dish. Still have room for the celery tuber.

12. Wash the tomatoes and halve them. Arrange them on the edge of the serving dish.

13.   Wash the radishes and halve them. Place them on the edge of the serving dish.

14.   Also, place the drained capers and olives on the edge of the serving dish.

15.   Arrange the celery tuber cubes next to the haricot

verts.

16.   Sprinkle salt and pepper to taste over the eggs, tuna, and vegetables.

17.   Serve with mayonnaise or mix in the mayonnaise.

Whole Grain Pasta With Meat Sauce

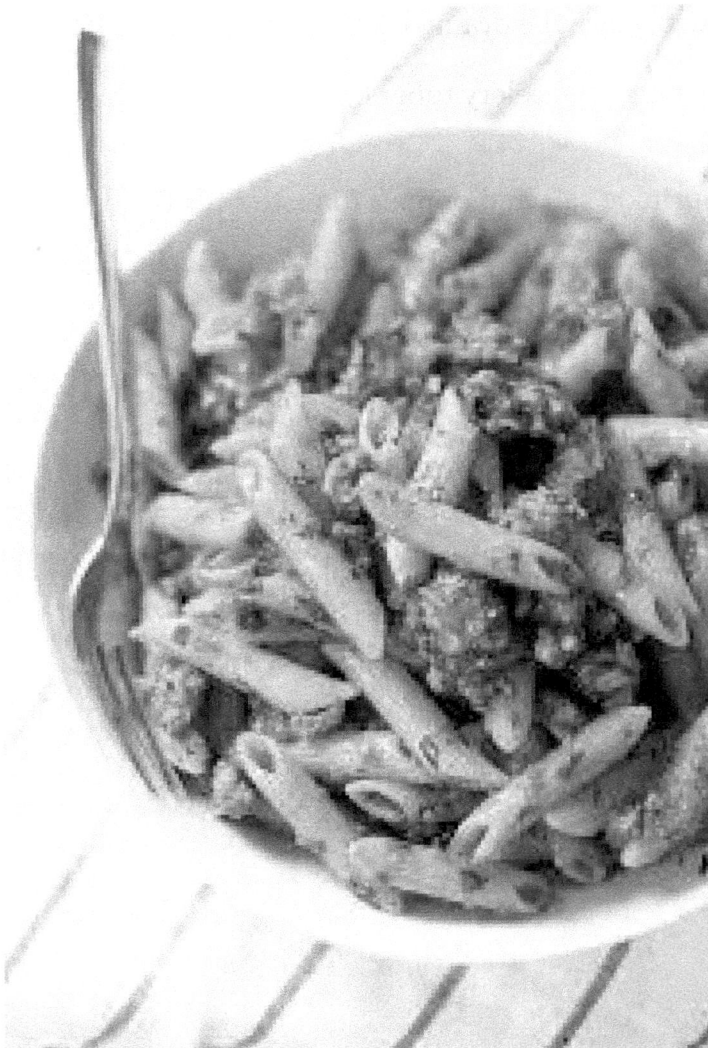

Prep time: 10 minutes

Cook time: 30 minutes

Servings: 6

Ingredients

- Whole-grain pasta – 1 pound

- Extra-lean ground beef – 1 pound

- Onion – 1, diced

- Garlic – 3 cloves, minced

- No-salt-added tomato sauce – 2 (8-ounce) cans

- Red wine – 1/3 cup

- Balsamic vinegar – 1 Tbsp.

- Dried basil - 1 tsp.

- Dried marjoram – ½ tsp.

- Dried oregano – ½ tsp.

- Dried red pepper flakes - ½ tsp.

- Dried thyme - ½ tsp.

- Freshly ground black pepper - ½ tsp.

Method

1.   Follow the direction on the package and cook the pasta. Omit the salt. Drain and set aside.

2.   Place onion, ground beef and garlic in a pan over medium heat. Stir-fry for 5 minutes, or until the beef has browned.
3.   Add remaining ingredients and stir to combine. Simmer, uncovered, for 10 minutes, stirring occasionally.
4.   Remove from heat and spoon over pasta.
5.   Serve.

Nutritional Facts Per Serving

Calories: 387

Fat: 5g

Carb: 58g

Protein: 27g

Sodium 65mg

Beef Tacos

Prep time: 10 minutes

Cook time: 20 minutes

Servings: 6

Ingredients

- Extra-lean ground beef – 1 pound

- Large onion – 1, chopped Garlic – 2 cloves, minced

- No-salt-added tomato sauce – 1 (8-ounce) can Low-sodium

- Worcestershire sauce – 2 tsp.
- Molasses - 1 Tbsp.

- Apple cider vinegar – 1 Tbsp.

- Ground cumin – 1 Tbsp.

- Ground sweet paprika – 1 Tbsp.

- Dried red pepper flakes - ½ tsp.

- Ground black pepper to taste

- Low-sodium taco shells – 1 package

- Chopped fresh cilantro - ¼ cup Tomato and lettuce of serving

Method

1.   Place the ground beef, onion, and garlic in a pan over medium heat.

2.   Stir-fry for 5 minutes or until the beef is browned.
3.   Lower heat to medium-low and add the Worcestershire sauce, tomato sauce, molasses, vinegar, cumin, red pepper flakes, paprika, and black pepper. Simmer, stirring frequently, about 10 minutes.

4.   Heat taco shells according to package directions. Set aside.
5.   Remove the sauté pan from the heat. Stir in cilantro.
6.   Divide evenly between the taco shells.
7.   Garnish with lettuce, tomato and serve.

Nutritional Facts Per Serving (2 tacos)

Calories: 255

Fat: 9g

Carb: 23g

Protein: 18g

Sodium 79mg

Dirty Rice

Prep time: 10 minutes

Cook time: 30 minutes

Servings: 4

Ingredients

- Extra-lean ground beef - ½ pound

- Large onion – 1, diced

- Celery – 2 stalks, diced

- Garlic – 2 cloves, minced

- Bell pepper – 1, diced

- Sodium-free beef bouillon granules - 1 tsp.

- Water - 1 cup

- Low-sodium Worcestershire sauce – 2 tsp.

- Dried thyme – 1 ½ tsp.

- Dried basil – 1 tsp.

- Dried marjoram - ½ tsp.

- Ground black pepper - ¼ tsp.

- Pinch ground cayenne pepper

- Scallions – 2, diced

- Cooked long-grain brown rice – 3 cups

Method

1.   In a pan, place the onion, ground beef, celery, and garlic. Stir-fry for 5 minutes or until beef is browned.

2.   Add beef bouillon, bell pepper, water, sauce, and herbs and stir to combine.
3.   Bring to a boil.
4.   Then reduce heat to low, and cover.
5.   Simmer for 20 minutes.
6.   Stir in the scallions and simmer, uncovered, for 3 minutes.
7.   Remove from heat. Add cooked rice and stir to combine.
8.   Serve.

Nutritional Facts Per Serving

Calories: 272

Fat: 4g

Carb: 41g

Protein: 16g

Sodium 92mg

Beef With Pea Pods

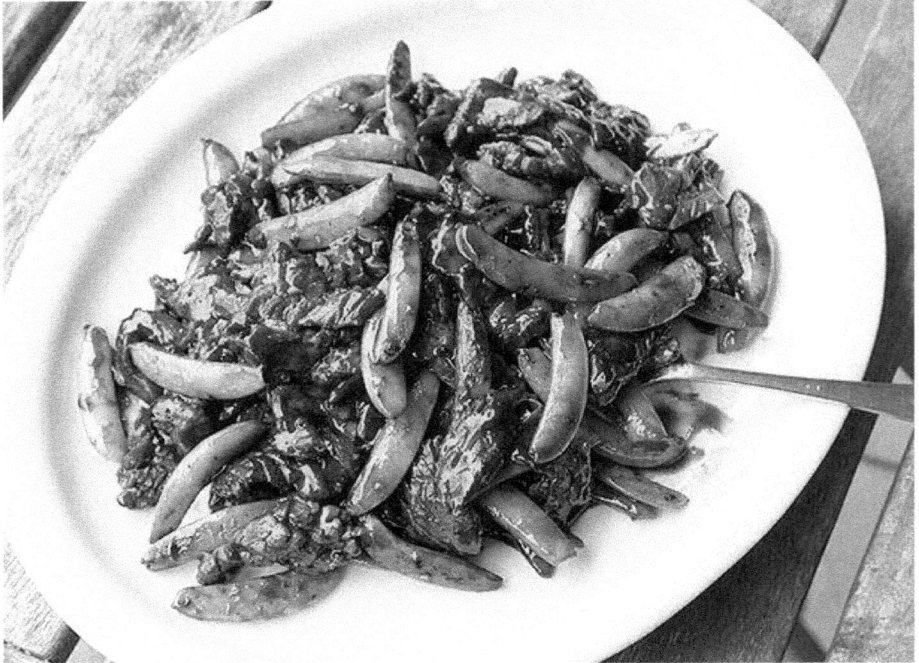

Prep time: 5 minutes

Cook time: 10 minutes

Servings: 4

Ingredients

- Thin beef steak – ¾ pound, sliced into thin strips

- Peanut oil – 1 Tbsp.

- Scallions – 3, sliced

- Garlic – 2 cloves, minced

- Minced fresh ginger – 2 tsp.

- Fresh pea pods – 4 cups, trimmed

- Homemade soy sauce – 3 Tbsp.

- Cooked brown rice – 4 cups

Method

1.   Heat the oil in a pan.

2.   Add the garlic, scallions, and ginger.
3.   Stir-fry for 30 seconds.
4.   Add the sliced beef and stir-fry for 5 minutes, or until beef has browned.
5.   Add pea pods and soy sauce and stir-fry for 3 minutes.
6.   Remove from heat.
7.   Serve with rice.

Homemade soy sauce

- Molasses – ¼ cup

- Unflavored rice wine vinegar – 3 Tbsp.

- Water – 1 Tbsp.

- Sodium-free beef bouillon granules – 1 tsp.

- Freshly ground black pepper - ½ tsp.

Method

1.   Mix everything in a saucepan and heat on low for 1 minute.

2.   Serve.

Nutritional Facts Per Serving

Calories: 466

Fat: 11g

Carb: 64g

Protein: 27g

Sodium 71mg

Whole-Grain Rotini With Ground Pork

Prep time: 10 minutes

Cook time: 25 minutes

Servings: 6

Ingredients

- Whole-grain rotini - 1 (13-ounce) package

- Lean ground pork – 1 pound

- Red onion – 1, chopped

- Garlic – 3 cloves, minced

- Bell pepper – 1, chopped

- Pumpkin puree – 1 cup Ground sage – 2 tsp.

- Ground rosemary – 1 tsp.

- Ground black pepper to taste

Method

1.   Cook the pasta (follow the package insturctions). Omit salt, drain and set aside.

2.   Heat a pan over medium heat. Add onion, garlic, and ground pork and sauté for 2 minutes.
3.   Add bell pepper and sauté for 5 minutes.
4.   Remove from heat. Add pasta to the pan along with remaining ingredients.
5.   Mix and serve.

Nutritional Facts Per Serving

Calories: 331

Fat: 7g

Carb: 45g

Protein: 23g

Sodium 48mg

Roasted Pork Loin With Herbs

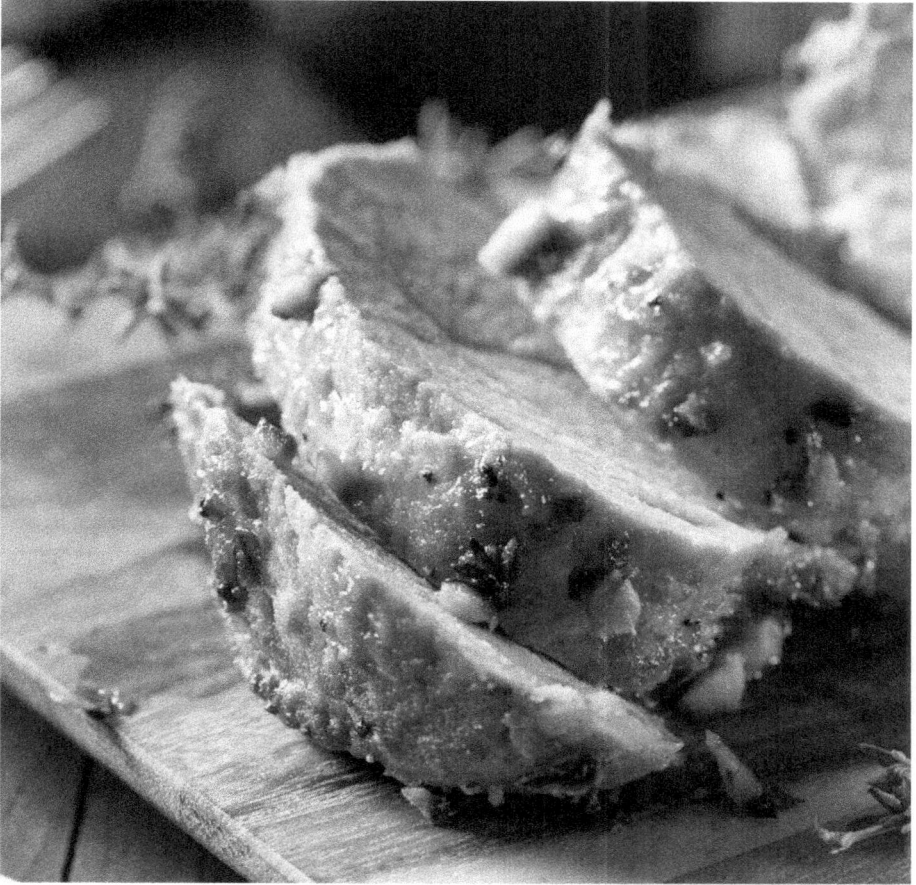

Prep time: 20 minutes

Cook time: 1 hour

Servings: 4

Ingredients

- Boneless pork loin roast – 2 lbs.

- Garlic – 3 cloves, minced Dried rosemary – 1 Tbsp.

- Dried thyme – 1 tsp.

- Dried basil – 1 tsp.

- Salt – ¼ tsp.

- Olive oil – ¼ cup

- White wine – ½ cup Pepper to taste

Method

1.   Preheat the oven to 350F.

2.   Crush the garlic with thyme, rosemary, basil, salt, and pepper, making a paste. Set aside.
3.   Use a knife to pierce meat several times.
4.   Press the garlic paste into the slits.
5.   Rub the meat with the rest of the garlic mixture and olive oil.
6.   Place pork loin into the oven, turning and basting with pan liquids, until the pork reaches 145F, about 1 hour. Remove the pork from the oven.
7.   Place the pan over heat and add white wine, stirring the brown bits on the bottom.
8.   Top roast with sauce.
9.   Serve.

Nutritional Facts Per Serving

Calories: 464

Fat: 20.7g

Carb: 2.4g

Protein: 59.6g

Sodium 279mg

Garlic Lime Pork Chops

Prep time: 20 minutes

Cook time: 10 minutes

Servings: 4

Ingredients

- Lean boneless pork chops – 4 (6-oz. each)

- Garlic – 4 cloves, crushed Cumin – ½ tsp.

- Chili powder - ½ tsp.

- Paprika - ½ tsp.

- Juice of ½ lime Lime zest – 1 tsp.

- Kosher salt - ¼ tsp.

- Fresh pepper to taste

Method

1.   In a bowl, season pork with cumin, chili powder, paprika, garlic salt, and pepper. Add lime juice and zest.

2.   Marinate the pork for 20 minutes.
3.   Line a broiler pan with foil.
4.   Place the pork chops on the broiler pan and broil for 5 minutes on each side or until browned.
5.   Serve.

Nutritional Facts Per Serving

Calories: 233

Fat: 13.2g

Carb: 4.3g

Protein: 25.5g

Sodium 592mg

Lamb Curry With Tomatoes And Spinach

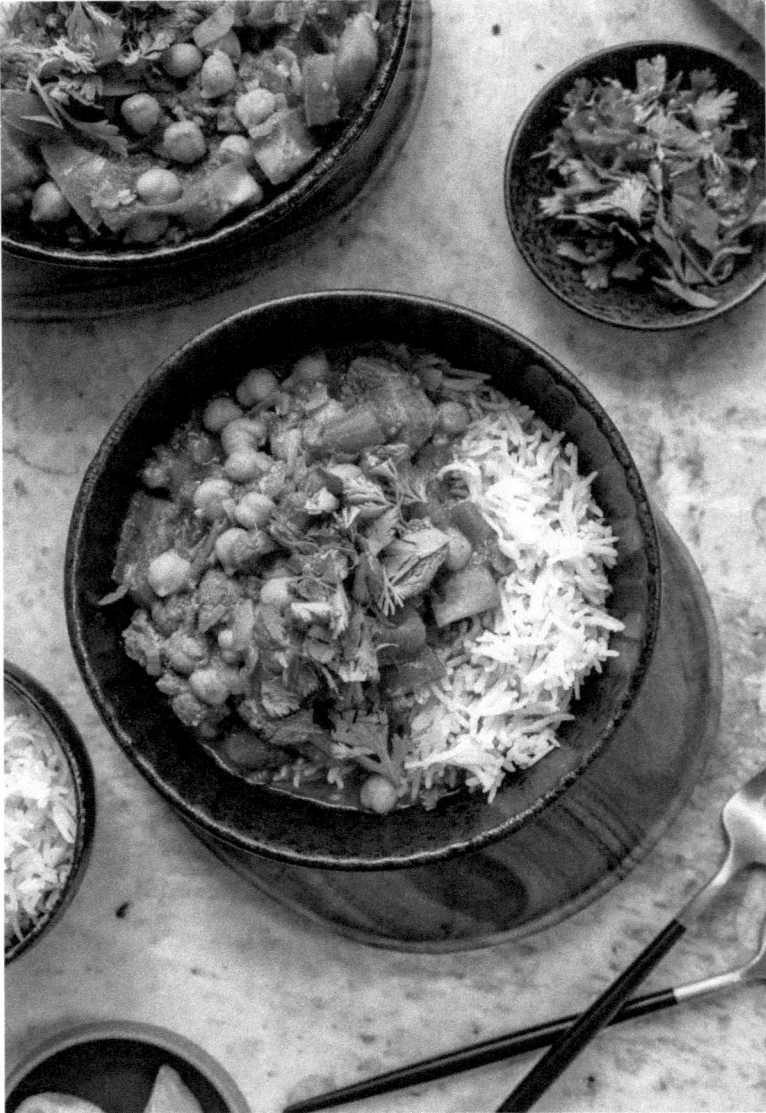

Prep time: 10 minutes

Cook time: 12 minutes

Servings: 4

Ingredients

- Olive oil – 1 tsp.

- Lean boneless lamb – 1 pound, sliced thinly Onion – 1, chopped

- Garlic – 3 cloves, minced Red bell pepper – 1, chopped Salt-free

- tomato paste – 2 Tbsp.
- Salt-free curry powder – 1 Tbsp.

- No-salt-added diced tomatoes – 1(15-ounce) can

- Fresh baby spinach – 10 ounces

- Low-sodium beef or vegetable broth - ½ cup

- Red wine – ¼ cup

- Chopped fresh cilantro – ¼ cup Ground black pepper to taste

Method

1.   Heat the oil in a pan.

2.   Add lamb and brown both sides, about 2 minutes.
3.   Add garlic, onion, and bell pepper. Stir-fry for 2 minutes. Stir in the curry powder and tomato paste.
4.   Add the tomatoes with juice, spinach, broth, and wine and stir to mix.
5.   Stir-fry for 3 to 4 minutes and lamb has cooked through.
6.   Remove from heat. Season with pepper and stir in cilantro.
7.   Serve.

Nutritional Facts Per Serving

Calories: 238

Fat: 7g

Carb: 14g

Protein: 27g

Sodium 167mg

Pomegranate-Marinated Leg Of Lamb

Prep time: 10 minutes

Cook time: 20 minutes

Servings: 6

Ingredients

For the marinate

- Bottled pomegranate juice - ½ cup

- Hearty red wine – ½ cup

- Ground cumin - 1 tsp.

- Dried oregano – 1 tsp.

- Crushed hot red pepper – ½ tsp.

- Garlic – 3 cloves, minced

For the lamb

- Boneless leg of lamb – 1 ¾ pound, butterflied and fat trimmed

- Kosher salt – ½ tsp.

- Olive oil spray

Method

1.   To make the marinade, whisk everything in a bowl and transfer to a zippered plastic bag.

2.   To prepare the lamb: add the lamb to the bag, press out the air, and close the bag. Marinate for 1 hour in the refrigerator.
3.   Preheat the broiler (8 inches from the source of heat).
4.   Remove the lamb from the marinade, blot with paper towels, but do not dry completely.
5.   Season with salt. Spray the broiler rack with oil.
6.   Place the lamb on the rack and broil, turning occasionally, about 20 minutes, or until lamb is browned and reaches 130F.
7.   Remove from heat, slice and serve with carving juices on top.

Nutritional Facts Per Serving

Calories: 273

Fat: 15g

Carb: 0g

Protein: 31g

Sodium 219mg

Beef Fajitas With Peppers

Prep time: 10 minutes

Cook time: 12 minutes

Servings: 6

Ingredients

- Olive oil – 2 tsp. plus more for the spray

- Sirloin steak – 1 pound, cut into bite-size pieces

- Red bell pepper – 1, chopped

- Green bell pepper – 1, chopped

- Red onion – 1, chopped

- Garlic - 2 cloves, minced

- DASH friendly Mexican seasoning – 1 Tbsp. (or any seasoning without salt)

- Boston lettuce leaves – 12 for serving Lime wedges or corn tortillas for serving

Method

Heat oil in a skillet.

Add half of the sirloin and cook until browned on both sides, about 2 minutes. Transfer to a plate.

Then repeat with the remaining sirloin.

Heat the 2 tsp. oil in the skillet.

Add onion, bell peppers, and garlic, cook and stir for 7 minutes or until tender.

Stir in the beef with any juices and the seasoning. Transfer to a plate.

Fill lettuce lead with beef mixture and drizzle lime juice on top.

Roll up and serve.

Nutritional Facts Per Serving

Calories: 231

Fat: 12g

Carb: 6g

Protein: 24g

Sodium 59mg

Pork Medallions With Herbs De Provence

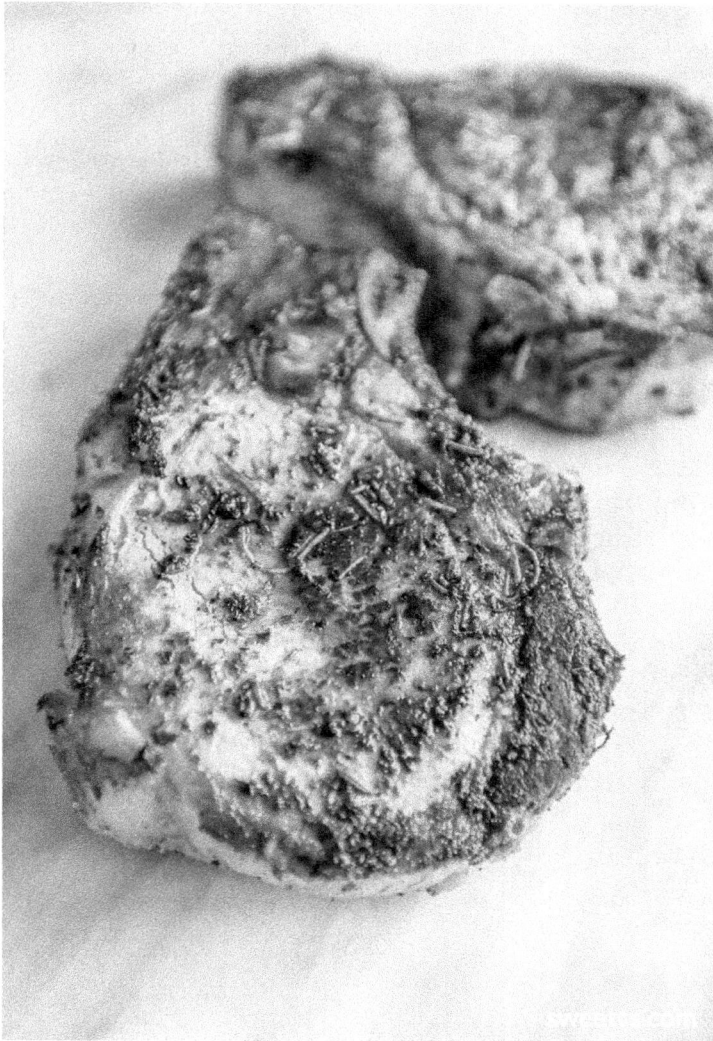

Prep time: 5 minutes

Cook time: 10 minutes

Servings: 2

Ingredients

- Pork tenderloin – 8 ounces, cut into 6 pieces (crosswise)

- Ground black pepper to taste Herbs de Provence – ½ tsp. Dry white wine – ¼ cup

Method

1. Season the pork with black pepper.

2. Place the pork between waxed paper sheets and roll with a rolling pin until about ¼ inch thick.
3. Cook the pork in a pan for 2 to 3 minutes on each side.
4. Remove from heat and season with the herb.
5. Place the pork on plates and keep warm.
6. Cook the wine in the pan until boiling. Scrape to get the brown bits from the bottom.
7. Serve pork with the sauce.

Nutritional Facts Per Serving

Calories: 120

Fat: 2g

Carb: 1g

Protein: 24g

Sodium 62mg

Baked Chicken

Prep time: 10 minutes

Cook time: 1 hour

Servings: 4

Ingredients

- Chicken – 3 to 4 pound, cut into parts Olive oil – 3 Tbsp.

- Thyme – ½ tsp.

- Sea salt – ¼ tsp.

- Ground black pepper

- Low-sodium chicken stock – ½ cup

Method

1.   Preheat the oven to 400F.

2.   Rub oil over chicken pieces. Sprinkle with salt, thyme, and pepper.

3.   Place chicken in the roasting pan.
4.   Bake in the oven for 30 minutes.
5.   Then lower the heat to 350F.

6.   Bake for 15 to 30 minutes more or until juice runs clear.
7.   Serve.

Nutritional Facts Per Serving

Calories: 550

Fat: 19g

Carb: 0g

Protein: 91g

Sodium 480mg

Orange Chicken And Broccoli Stir-Fry

Prep time: 10 minutes

Cook time: 15 minutes

Servings: 4

Ingredients

- Olive oil – 1 Tbsp.

- Chicken breast – 1 pound, boneless and skinless, cut into strips Orange juice – 1/3 cup Homemade soy sauce - 2 Tbsp.

- Cornstarch – 2 tsp.

- Broccoli – 2 cups, cut into small pieces Snow peas – 1 cup

- Cabbage – 2 cups, shredded Brown rice – 2 cups, cooked Sesame seeds – 1 Tbsp.

Method

1.   Combine the orange juice, soy sauce, and corn starch in a bowl. Set aside.

2.   Heat oil in a pan. Add chicken.

3.   Stir-fry until the chicken is golden brown on all sides, about 5 minutes.
4.   Add snow peas, cabbage, broccoli, and sauce mixture.
5.   Continue to stir-fry for 8 minutes or until vegetables are tender but still crisp.

Nutritional Facts Per Serving

Calories: 340

Fat: 8g

Carb: 35g

Protein: 28g

Sodium 240mg

Mediterranean Lemon Chicken And Potatoes

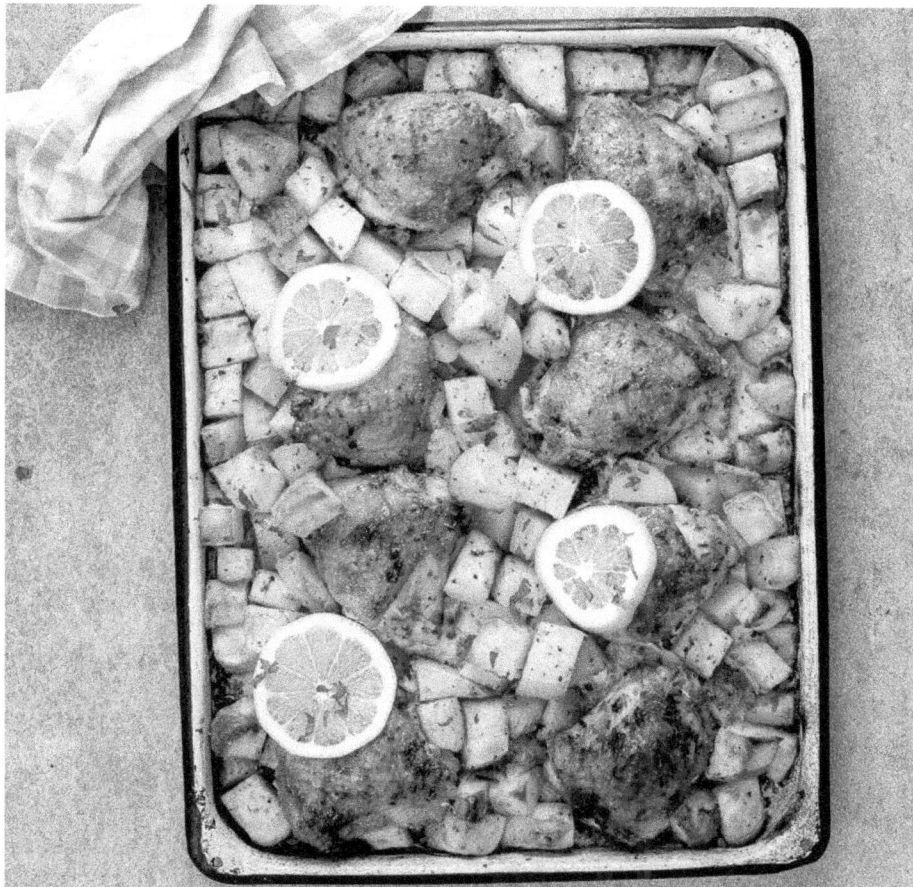

Prep time: 10 minutes

Cook time: 30 minutes

Servings: 4

Ingredients

- Chicken breast – 1 ½ pound, skinless and boneless, cut into 1-inch cubes

- Yukon Gold potatoes – 1 pound, cut into cubes

- Onion – 1, chopped

- Red pepper – 1, chopped

- Low-sodium vinaigrette – ½ cup

- Lemon juice – ¼ cup Oregano – 1 tsp.

- Garlic powder – ½ tsp.

- Chopped tomato – ½ cup

- Ground black pepper to taste

Method

8.   Preheat oven to 400F.

2.   Except for the tomatoes, mix everything in a bowl.
3.   On 4 aluminum foils, place an equal amount of chicken and potato mixture. Fold to make packets.

4.   Bake at 400F for 30 minutes. Open packets.
5.   Top with chopped tomatoes.
6.   Season with black pepper to taste.

Nutritional Facts Per Serving

Calories: 320

Fat: 4g

Carb: 34g

Protein: 43g

Sodium 420mg

Tandoori Chicken

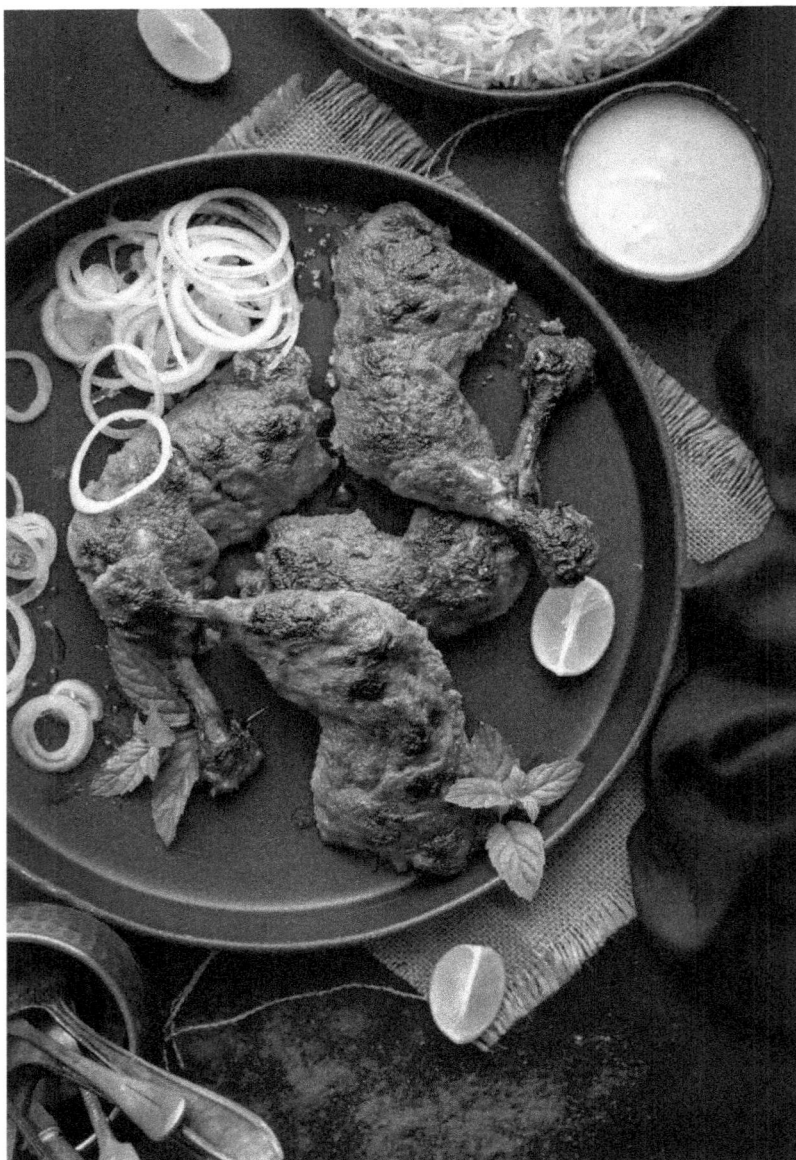

Prep time: 10 minutes

Cook time: 20 minutes

Servings: 6

Ingredients

- Nonfat yogurt – 1 cup, plain

- Lemon juice – ½ cup Garlic – 5 cloves, crushed Paprika – 2 Tbsp.

- Curry powder – 1 tsp.

- Ground ginger – 1 tsp.

- Red pepper flakes – 1 tsp.

- Chicken breasts – 6, skinless and boneless, cut into 2-inch chunks Wooden skewers – 6, soaked in water

Method

8.   Preheat the oven to 400F.

2.   In a bowl, combine lemon juice, yogurt, garlic, and spices. Blend well.
3.   Divide chicken and thread onto skewers. Place skewers in a baking dish.
4.   Pour half of the yogurt mixture onto chicken. Cover and marinate in the refrigerator for 20 minutes
5.   Spray a baking dish with cooking spray.

6.   Place chicken skewers in the pan and coat with the remaining ½ of yogurt marinade.

7.   Bake in the oven until chicken is cooked, about 15 to 20 minutes.

8.   Serve with veggies or brown rice.

Nutritional Facts Per Serving

Calories: 175

Fat: 2g

Carb: 8g

Protein: 30g

Sodium 105mg

Orange-Rosemary Roasted Chicken

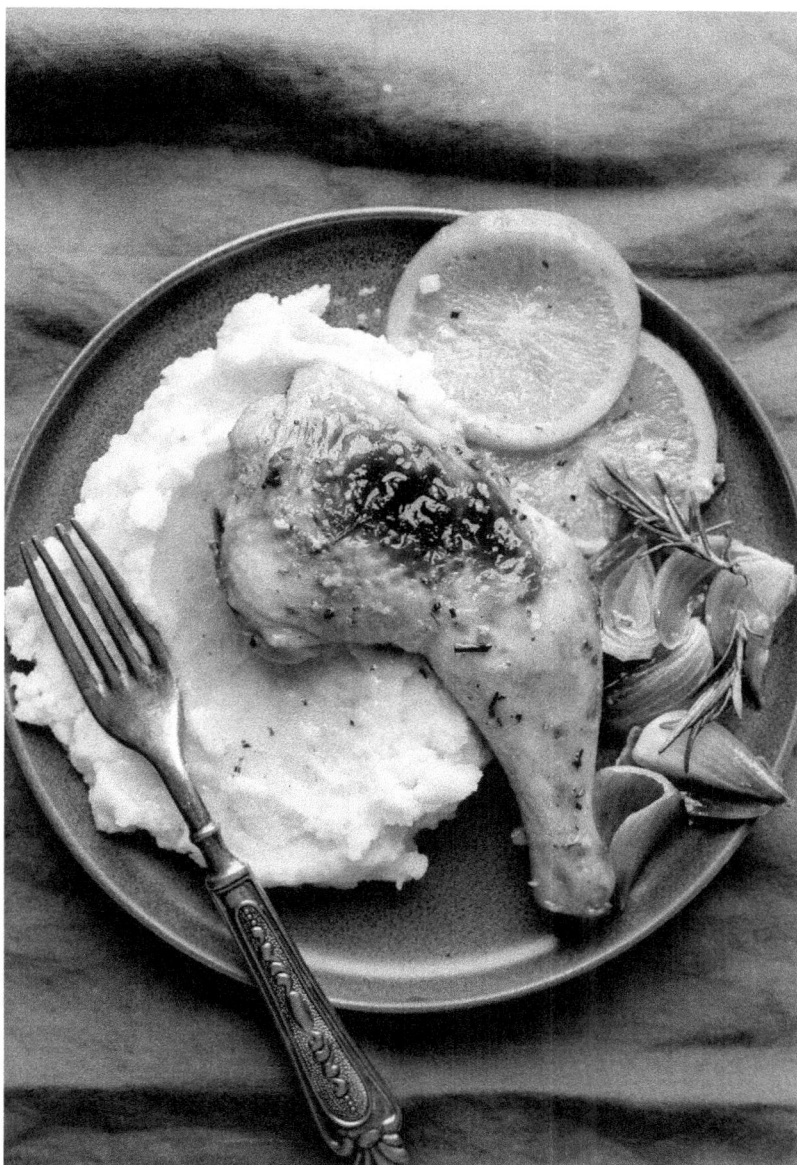

Prep time: 10 minutes

Cook time: 45 minutes

Servings: 6

Ingredients

- Chicken breast halves – 3, skinless, bone-in, each 8 ounces
  Chicken legs with thigh pieces – 3, skinless, bone-in, each 8 ounces

- Garlic cloves – 2, minced Extra-virgin olive oil – 1 ½ tsp.

- Fresh rosemary – 3 tsp.

- Ground black pepper – 1/8 tsp.

- Orange juice – ½ cup

Method

1.   Preheat oven at 450F. Grease a baking pan with cooking spray.

2.   Rub chicken with garlic, then with oil. Sprinkle with pepper and rosemary.
3.   Place the chicken pieces in the baking dish.
4.   Pour the orange juice.
5.   Cover and bake for 30 minutes, then flip the chicken with tongs and cook 10 to 15 minutes more or until browned. Baste the chicken with the pan juice from time to time.
6.   Serve chicken with pan juice.

Nutritional Facts Per Serving

Calories: 204

Fat: 8g

Carb: 2g

Protein: 31g

Sodium 95mg

Honey Crusted Chicken

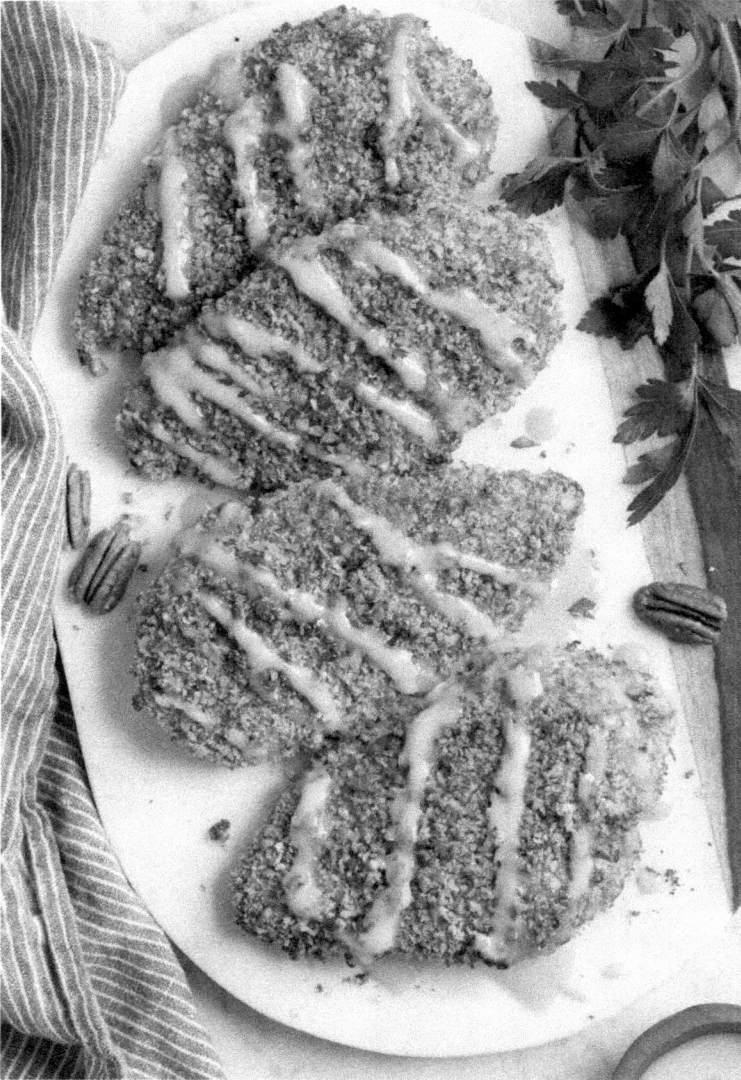

Prep time: 10 minutes

Cook time: 25 minutes

Servings: 2

Ingredients

- Saltine crackers – 8, (2-inch square each) crushed Paprika – 1 tsp.

- Chicken breasts – 2, boneless, skinless (4-ounce each)

- Honey – 4 tsp.

- Cooking spray to grease a baking sheet

Method

1. Preheat the oven to 375F.

2. In a bowl, mix crushed crackers and paprika. Mix well.
3. In another bowl, add honey and chicken. Coat well.
4. Add to the cracker mixture and coat well.
5. Place the chicken in the prepared baking sheet.
6. Bake for 20 to 25 minutes.
7. Serve.

Nutritional Facts Per Serving

Calories: 219

Fat: 3g

Carb: 21g

Protein: 27g

Sodium 187mg

Italian Chicken And Vegetable

Prep time: 10 minutes

Cook time: 45 minutes

Servings: 1

Ingredients

Chicken breast

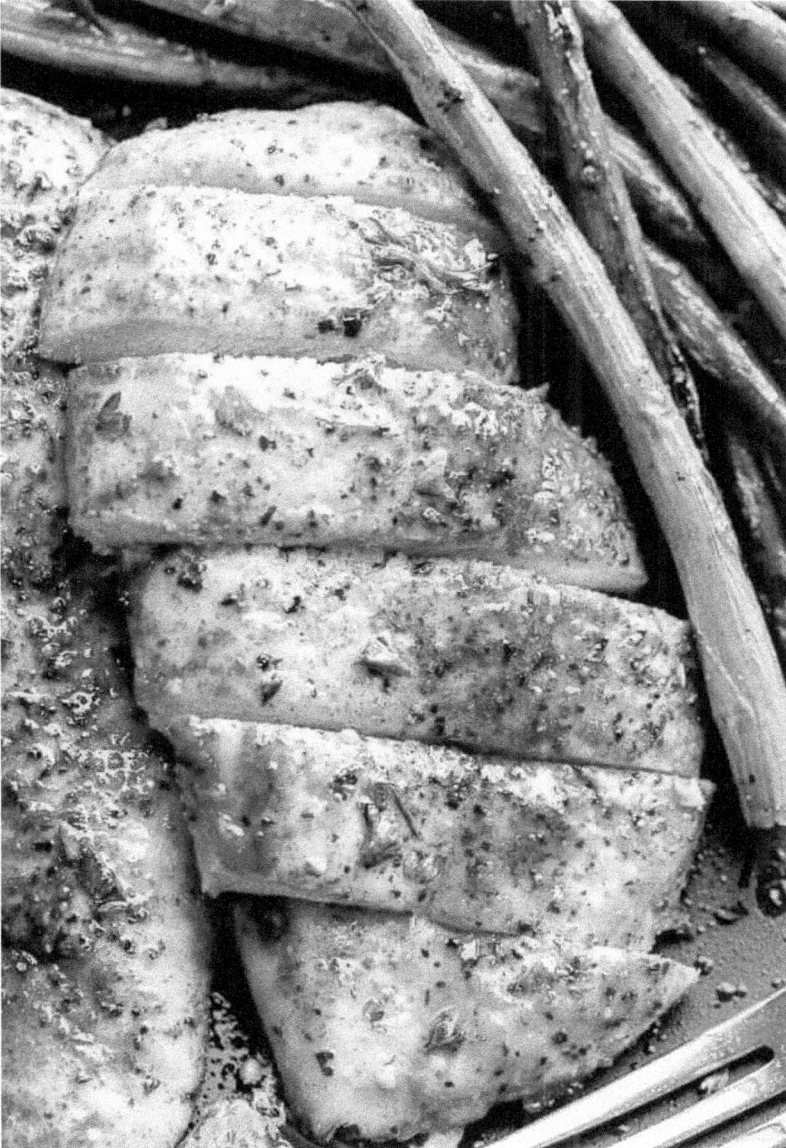

- 1 skinless, boneless (3 ounces)

- Diced zucchini – ½ cup

- Diced potato – ½ cup

- Diced onion – ¼ cup

- Sliced baby carrots – ¼ cup

- Sliced mushrooms – ¼ cup

- Garlic powder – 1/8 tsp.

- Italian seasoning – ¼ tsp.

Method

1.   Preheat oven to 350F.

2.   Grease a parchment paper with cooking spray.
3.   On the foil, add chicken, top mushrooms, carrots, onion, potato, and zucchini. Sprinkle with Italian seasoning and garlic powder.
4.   Fold the foil to make a packet.
5.   Place the packet on a cookie sheet.
6.   Bake until chicken and vegetables are tender, about 45 minutes.

7.   Serve.

Nutritional Facts Per Serving

Calories: 207

Fat: 2.5g

Carb: 23g

Protein: 23g

Sodium 72mg

www.ingramcontent.com/pod-product-compliance
Lightning Source LLC
Chambersburg PA
CBHW062118040426
42336CB00041B/1899